Sanger/Bross Clinical Management of Child Abuse and Neglect

Clinical Management of Child Abuse and Neglect

A Guide for the Dental Professional

Edited by

Roger G. Sanger, D.D.S., M.S.Ed.
Professor of Pediatric Dentistry and Oral Medicine
School of Dentistry, Health Sciences Center
University of Colorado, Denver.

Donald C. Bross, J.D., Ph.D.
Assistant Professor in Pediatrics (Family Law)
School of Medicine, Health Sciences Center
University of Colorado, Denver.

quintessence books

Quintessence Publishing Co., Inc. 1984
Chicago, London, Berlin, Rio de Janeiro and Tokyo

Library of Congress Cataloging in Publication Data
Main entry under title:

Clinical management of child abuse and neglect.

1. Mouth—Wounds and injuries. 2. Face—Wounds and injuries. 3. Battered child syndrome. 4. Pedodontics. 5. Dental jurisprudence. I. Sanger, Roger G. II. Bross, Donald C. [DNLM: 1. Child abuse. 2. Maxillofacial injuries—Therapy. 3. Forensic dentistry. WA 320 C641]
RK493.C55C55 1983 617′.522044 83-23038
ISBN 0-86715-128-5

quintessence books

Composition: Typographic Sales, St. Louis
Printing and binding: BookCrafters, Chelsea, MI
Printed in U.S.A.

Contributors

JoAnn Avila, M.S.W.
Clinical Social Worker
Child Protection Team
School of Medicine
University of Colorado
Health Sciences Center
Denver

Paul S. Casamassimo, D.D.S., M.S.
Associate Professor and Chairman
Department of Growth and Development
School of Dentistry
University of Colorado
Health Sciences Center
Denver

Peter K. Domoto, D.D.S., M.P.H.
Associate Professor and Chairman
Department of Pedodontics
School of Dentistry
University of Washington
Health Sciences Center
Seattle

Edward J. Goldson, M.D.
Assistant Professor of Pediatrics
School of Medicine
University of Colorado
Health Sciences Center
Director of the Newborn Follow-Up Program
Children's Hospital
Denver

Candace A. Grosz, M.A.
Information Director
The C. Henry Kempe National Center for Prevention and Treatment of Child Abuse and Neglect
Denver

David L. Kerns, M.D.
Director of Ambulatory Services
Children's Hospital Medical Center
Oakland

Lowell J. Levine, D.D.S.
Forensic Odontologist
County of Nassau
Clinical Associate Professor of Forensic Medicine
School of Medicine
New York University
New York

Howard L. Needleman, D.M.D.
Assistant Clinical Professor of Pediatric Dentistry
School of Dental Medicine
Harvard University
Dentist-in-Chief
Children's Hospital Medical Center
Boston

Arthur J. Nowak, D.M.D., M.A.
Professor of Pedodontics
College of Dentistry
University of Iowa
Iowa City

Robert F. Primosch, D.D.S., M.S.
Associate Professor of Pedodontics
College of Dentistry
University of Oklahoma
Health Sciences Center
Oklahoma City

Kristin F. Robbins, D.D.S.
Assistant Clinical Professor of Applied Dentistry
School of Dentistry
University of Colorado
Health Sciences Center
Denver

Barton D. Schmitt, M.D.
Associate Professor of Pediatrics and Director of Child Protection Team
School of Medicine
University of Colorado
Health Sciences Center
Denver

Richard S. Sobel, D.D.S.
Director of Dentistry
Children's Hospital Medical Center of Northern California
Oakland

Norman D. Sperber, D.D.S.
Forensic Odontologist
County of San Diego
San Diego

Ray E. Stewart, D.M.D., M.S.
Professor of Pediatric Dentistry and Pediatrics (Medical Genetics)
University of California at Los Angeles
Harbor General Hospital
Torrance

Table of Contents

To children abused or neglected
and to people who care

Forewords

This book fills an important void in child abuse literature. As health professionals, dentists—like physicians—are included among those required by state laws to report suspected cases of child abuse. An interesting but little-known fact is that traumatic oral and facial injuries may be the first presented finding, and the dentist may be the first health care provider who has access to the child or adolescent involved in abuse. This first comprehensive book in the field, aside from giving an overview of the problem, deals with the subject beyond the most obvious oral facial injuries by including material that to some dentists may be surprising.

Clinical Management of Child Abuse and Neglect should be read by all dentists, especially by those who see children and adolescents in their daily practice.

C. Henry Kempe, M.D.
Director-Emeritus
C. Henry Kempe National Center for Prevention
and Treatment of Child Abuse and Neglect, Denver
Professor of Pediatrics and Microbiology
University of Colorado Health Sciences Center
School of Medicine, Denver

Many years ago, C. Henry Kempe, M.D., the man most responsible for all of us having an intense commitment to this field, told me that most of his malpractice suits as chairman of pediatrics came from cases seen in the emergency room at night. As he put it, the problem was that the least experienced personnel (first-year interns) were in the most vulnerable positions. ''They don't know what they don't know, and the pressure is too great not to admit or ask for help,'' Kempe said. He subsequently put second-year residents on from 6 p.m. to 8 a.m., and the number of suits dropped.

Why begin an introduction to this book for dental health professionals with that story? First, dental health professionals are among the most likely, along with emergency-room professionals, to deal with traumatic injury to children. Therefore, awareness of abuse as an *etiology* for trauma is important.

Secondly, the nature of dental therapy allows more time to think about how to proceed. I worry about emergency room professionals who by their very choice of career may be saying they don't want ongoing relationships with people and who, in my experience, are reluctant to get involved in these cases. Dental health professionals are different. They have ongoing relationships with their patients, and they have the time, although never enough, to explore the psychological problems of their patients.

That does not mean dental professionals have to solve the problem; help is just a phone call away. But involvement is necessary if we are to protect and nurture the small percentage, yet large number, of children in our society who are emotionally abandoned by their parents.

This book will help dental professionals learn what they need to know about child abuse and neglect. The next step involves looking around. Not only will professionals find what is described here, but the boundaries of their practice will transcend their four walls. Then they can contribute to a second, enlarged edition of this book.

Richard D. Krugman, M.D.
Director
C. Henry Kempe National Center for Prevention and Treatment of Child Abuse and Neglect, Denver

Preface

Interdisciplinary cooperation offers major opportunities for new knowledge, new techniques, and better management of patient care by the dental profession. In turn, the dental profession can contribute greatly to other fields. This text highlights the dental profession's accomplishments and achievements in one of many available interdisciplinary health care arenas: health care of children worldwide, especially as it relates to parenting and parent-child relationships.

We hope that dental professionals, irrespective of nationality or discipline, will find this a useful introduction and general reference on the problems of child abuse and neglect. Health care of children must transcend geographic and professional barriers. Many of the contributors to this text have been leaders in the dissemination of knowledge about child abuse and neglect and its implications for dental practice, education, and research, both nationally and internationally.

Innumerable institutions deserve recognition and thanks for their support of this book, including those who follow:

The National Center on Child Abuse and Neglect, Washington, D.C., for its administrative and financial support for a major conference for dental professionals on child abuse and neglect, which facilitated identification and cooperation of many of the authors.

The C. Henry Kempe National Center for the Prevention and Treatment of Child Abuse and Neglect, Denver, Colorado, for the support of its faculty and staff, especially Ms. Isabel Falk.

The University of Colorado Health Sciences Center School of Dentistry for the support of its faculty and continuing education staff, especially Mr. Denver Maine.

The advisory committee members, speakers, and participants for their support of the National Conference on Implications of Child Abuse and Neglect for the Dental Profession held June 8–9, 1981, in Denver, Colorado, which served as the genesis of this text.

The contributors of this text for their dedication and cooperation.

The Quintessence Publishing Company, Inc., for insuring the availability of these collected materials to the dental profession.

Our devoted secretaries without whose help these manuscripts would not have been typed and processed for submission.

With gratitude we recognize that our most personal support and understanding has continued to come from our wives and children, a reminder of how much families mean to all of us.

Roger G. Sanger/Donald C. Bross

Chapter 1

Professional Responsibility in Child Abuse and Neglect

Roger G. Sanger

Introduction

Numerous editorials have appeared in national dental journals addressing the professional responsibilities in child abuse and neglect and citing the need for continuing professional education (Laskin, 1973; Teuscher, 1974; Woods, 1975; Laskin, 1978; Scholle, 1978; Teuscher, 1979). Articles have appeared in national dental auxiliary journals with similar emphases (ten Bensel et al., 1977; Benusis, 1978; Bowen, 1980; Kenney, 1981b), and in *New Dentist,* the national dental student journal, with dedication of an entire volume (Seaman, 1981; Curtin, 1981; Johnson, 1981; Kenney, 1981a).

Resolution 97H of the 1979 House of Delegates of the American Dental Association encourages members to be more mindful of their responsibilities and asks the Council on Dental Practice to disseminate information on the professional and legal aspects of child abuse. The Bureau of Economic and Behavioral Research of the American Dental Association prepared a report on these responsibilities for the council that is now available from the association (ADA, 1980). Two recent surveys of dentists in the United States cite unawareness by dentists and the need for expanded professional education. In a national survey of 246 pediatric dentists, only nine percent had ever filed a report of child abuse. Alarmingly, seven percent cited some explanation to indicate they would never make reports. Almost 90 percent, however, were aware of the problem and said they would make a report of evidence-suggested abuse (Malecz, 1979). In a survey of 1,332 dentists in one state, less than 45 percent of dentists were aware of their responsibilities. Pediatric dentists and oral surgeons were more aware and involved (Becker et al., 1978). Despite professional ethics and legislative mandates, it appears that dentists have either an unawareness of or lack of compliance with professional responsibilities. Statistics reveal that more than half of all cases of reported child abuse involve craniofacial trauma (Becker et al., 1978). It would seem likely, then, that dentists treat children who may be victims of child abuse. Hopefully, the plethora of information on the dentist's responsibilities in identification, treatment, prevention, and in the reporting of child abuse and neglect will address this unawareness. Lack of compliance, although remaining an individual issue, may decrease as awareness increases.

The Dentist's Responsibilities

The responsibilities of the dental professional in child abuse and neglect include *identification* of the abuse or neglect, *treatment* of the child's injury or neglect, and *prevention* of further abuse or neglect, with complete *reporting* to appropriate agencies required.

Although they may sound simple when stated, these responsibilities are actually very complex. The dental professional often faces an insurmountable dilemma when confronted with suspicion of child abuse or neglect in his/her practice. It is the intent of this book to remove barriers preventing the dental professional from fulfilling these responsibilities with confidence and pride. The dental professional is an important member of the health care delivery system, a system which continues to expand its parameters, adding to its complexity. It is vital to the mainstream of this system that the dental professional understand, accept, and fulfill his/her professional responsibilities.

Failure to Respond

The dental professional who fails to fulfill the professional responsibilities in child abuse and neglect may do so for a variety of reasons. These may include the following (ten Bensel and King, 1975; Becker et al., 1978; Davis et al., 1979; Malecz, 1979):

- Lack of knowledge of child abuse and neglect
- Difficulties in diagnosis
- Fear of legal involvement
- Effect on practice
- Fear of confrontation
- Lack of confidence in the social service system
- Isolation from social service or health agencies
- Lack of confidence in parents and child
- Variation in acceptable definitions
- Indifference to family matters
- Disruption of dentist/patient relationships
- Fear of physical and/or verbal reprisals

Dentists who fulfilled their responsibilities in suspected cases of child abuse or neglect reported minimal effects on their practices. With proper handling of communication with parents and agencies even these minimal effects could be avoided (Davis et al., 1979).

Profile of Child Abuse

It is estimated that there are approximately one million incidents of physical child abuse yearly, resulting in approximately 2,000 deaths (Kearns, 1979). This does not include emotional abuse, sexual abuse, or neglect. It is thought that for every case of physical abuse reported, a hundred may go undiagnosed or unreported (Gil, 1970).

The number of new cases reported each year creates an inverse pyramid effect when added to cases already under management and treatment, some spanning many years. Five percent of the many physically abused children who are returned to their parents or guardians without intervention are later killed or die and 35 percent are seriously reinjured (Schmitt and Kempe, 1975). The sequelae of abuse or nonaccidental injury to a developing child is now recognized as one of the major causes of developmental disabilities (Martin et al., 1974). The mortality rate from abuse of children one to six months of age is second only to the sudden infant death syndrome, and in one- to five-year-olds, second only to accidents (McNeese and Hebeler, 1977).

An Interdisciplinary Approach

Certainly the dental profession is indebted to its colleagues in the health, allied health, and legal professions for information pertinent to the general aspects in the prevention and treatment of child abuse and neglect. However, this information is devoid of data and recommendations on the issues and problems faced by the dental profession.

These issues and problems specific to the dental profession must be addressed by more than just the dental profession. As is the case with issues and problems faced by the medical, nursing, legal, and educational professions, dental issues must be addressed by an interdisciplinary representatation of all these professions. Child dental abuse and dental neglect are definitely part of the entire spectrum of child abuse and neglect. The dental profession must be informed of health, social, and legislative aspects of child abuse and neglect. Likewise, the other professions must realize that child dental/oral/facial abuse and dental care neglect is a definite reality in child abuse and neglect and needs the same research, investigation, educational material, and clinical service protocols/manuals developed specifically for these issues and problems as has been accomplished in other disciplines.

Continuing professional education for dentists and inclusion of dentists on child protection teams can substantially increase reported cases of suspected child abuse by the dental profession (Blain et al., 1979). Interdisciplinary approaches to child abuse and neglect are paramount.

A National Conference

On June 8–9, 1981, the University of Colorado Health Sciences Center Schools of Dentistry and Medicine and the National Center for the Prevention and Treatment of Child Abuse and Neglect sponsored—under the direction of Roger G. Sanger, D.D.S., and Donald C. Bross, J.D., Ph.D., and with the support from the National Center on Child Abuse and Neglect—a national conference in Denver on the implications of child abuse and neglect on dental education and practice. Speakers representing various disciplines of pediatrics, psychiatry, forensic pathology, family law, social services, forensic odontology, pediatric dentistry, oral surgery, and general dentistry delivered presentations on child abuse and neglect. Numerous participants representing the academies of these disciplines and numerous editors of professional journals were in attendance. The proceedings of that conference served as the genesis of this book.

References

American Dental Association (ADA), Council on Dental Practice: The Dentist's Responsibility in Recognizing and Reporting Child Abuse. Chicago: ADA, 1980.

Becker, D.B.; Needleman, H.L.; and Kotelchuck, M.: Child Abuse and Dentistry: Orofacial Trauma and Its Recognition by Dentists. J. Am. Dent. Assoc. 97:24, 1978.

Benusis, K.: Child Abuse: What the Dentist Should Know. Dent. Assist. 47:22, 1978.

Blain, S.M.; Winegarden, T.; Barber, T.K.; and Sognnaes, R.F.: Child Abuse and Neglect II—Dentistry's Role. IADR (ABS) 1105, J. Dent. Res. 58:367, 1979.

Bowen, P.L.: Child Neglect Identification: The Hygienist and Child Advocacy. Dent. Hyg. 54:71–73, 1980.

Curtin, C.: Can You Be Touched By Child Abuse. New Dent. 11:8, 1981.

Davis, G.R.; Domoto, P.K.; and Levy, R.L.: The Dentist's Role in Child Abuse and Neglect—Issues, Identification and Management. J. Dent. Child. 46:185–192, 1979.

Gil, D.: Violence Against Children: Physical Abuse in the United States. Cambridge, Mass.: Harvard University Press, 1970.

Johnson, D.M.: Child Abuse and the Law. New Dent. 11:15, 1981.

Kearns, D.: Child Abuse and Neglect: The Pediatrician's Role. JCE Pediatr. 21:11, 1979.

Kenney, J. P.: Child Abuse and the Dental Health Professional. New Dent. 11:17, 1981a.

Kenney, J.P.: Recognizing Child Abuse and Neglect—A Professional Responsibility. Quint. J. 3:269, 1981b.

Laskin, D.M.: The Battered Child Syndrome. J. Oral Surg. 31:903, 1973.

Laskin, D.M.: The Recognition of Child Abuse. J. Oral Surg. 36:349, 1978.

Malecz, R.E.: Child Abuse: Its Relationship to Pedodontics: A Survey. J. Dent. Child. 46:193–194, 1979.

McNeese, M.C. and Hebeler, J.R.: The Abused Child—A Clinical Approach to Identification and Management. Clin. Symp. 29(5):1–36, 1977.

Schmitt, B.D. and Kempe, C.H.: Neglect and Abuse of Children. In Vaughan, V.C. and McKay, R.J. (ed.) Nelson Textbook of Pediatrics. (10th ed.). Philadelphia: W.B. Saunders Co., 1975.

Scholle, R.H.: Sobs in Silence? J. Am. Dent. Assoc. 97:153–154, 1978.

Seaman, B.: "He Cried when They Sent Him Home." New Dent. 11:4, 1981.

ten Bensel, R.W. and King, K.: Neglect and Abuse of Children: Historical Aspects, Identification and Management. J. Dent. Child. 42:348, 1975.

ten Bensel, R.W.; King, K.; and Bastein, S.A.: Child Abuse and Neglect: History, Identification and Reporting. Dent. Hyg. 51:119–125, 1977.

Teuscher, G.W.: The Battered Child: A Social Enigma. J. Dent. Child. 41:335, 1974.

Teuscher, G.W.: It is Our Problem Too. J. Dent. Child. 46:184, 1979.

Woods, W.: Expanding our Responsibility. J. Dent. Child. 42:86, 1975.

Chapter 2

Child Abuse and Neglect: Types, Epidemiology, and Characteristics

Barton D. Schmitt

Introduction

Much has happened in our society since Dr. Kempe in 1961 coined the term "battered child syndrome" to describe children with numerous unexplained bruises, fractures, and head injuries. Today, when a "battered child" is encountered, we know our community detection and treatment systems have failed. Our goal today should be to recognize the many forms of child abuse at the earliest stages possible, before any permanent damage has occurred, and to refer these families for needed services. Eight subtypes of child abuse and neglect (Table 2-1) will be discussed by epidemiology and characteristic. Dentists are more likely to encounter physical abuse, sexual abuse, health care neglect, and safety neglect. Approximately one to two percent of children are abused or neglected. The incidence of each type in 1980 is recorded in Table 2-2.

Table 2-1 Types of child abuse and neglect

Physical abuse	Intentional drugging or poisoning	Emotional abuse and neglect
Sexual abuse	Health (medical) care neglect	Physical neglect
Failure to thrive	Safety neglect	Educational neglect

Types of Child Abuse

Physical Abuse

Physical abuse or nonaccidental trauma can be defined as injuries inflicted by a caretaker. Physical abuse is probably the most important subtype of child maltreatment because without intervention and services it is potentially fatal. Often the injury stems from an angry attempt of the caretaker to punish the child for misbehavior. Sometimes it is an uncontrolled lashing out at a child who happens to

Table 2-2 Incidence of child abuse and neglect in the United States for 1980 by type by substantiated reports*

Type	Number of children reported by type	Percent
Physical abuse	207,600	31.8
Sexual abuse	44,700	6.8
Failure to thrive	26,000	4.0
Intentional poisoning	not specified	—
Health (medical) care neglect	56,000	8.7
Safety neglect	not specified	—
Emotional abuse and neglect	171,400	26.3
Physical neglect	51,100	7.8
Educational neglect	181,500	27.8

*National Study of the Incidence and Severity of Child Abuse and Neglect, May 1, 1979, to April 30, 1980. Total substantiated cases: 652,000 or 10.5 per 1,000 incidences. Some children had multiple types of maltreatment.

be in the caretaker's way when some unrelated crisis occurs. Table 2-3 lists the characteristics most commonly encountered when interviewing abusive caretakers.

Physical trauma can be rated as *mild* (a few bruises, welts, scratches, cuts, scars), *moderate* (numerous bruises, minor burns, a single fracture), or *severe* (large burn, central nervous system injury, abdominal injury, multiple fractures, other life-threatening injury). Physically abused children are often young children.

Since physical punishment is commonplace in our society, physicians and dentists need guidelines as to when corporal punishment is excessive and therefore representative of physical abuse. Corporal punishment that causes bruises or leads to an injury that requires medical or dental treatment is outside the range of normal punishment. Bruising implies hitting without restraint. A few bruises explained in the name of discipline can easily proceed into a more serious injury the next time. Even when there are no signs of injury, an incident that includes hitting with a closed fist or kicking the child represents physical abuse. All of the preceding examples of corporal punishment should be reported to the appropriate agencies so that these families can learn safer ways of managing children and their behavior.

Reasonable physical punishment is not illegal. For those parents or caretakers who wish to use physical discipline techniques, certain guidelines for acceptable procedure should be discussed. First, the parent or caretaker should only utilize the hand. Striking a child with a blunt instrument can interfere with the adult's ability to titrate the amount of force applied. Paddles and belts commonly cause bruises that may not have been intended. Second, the child should only be struck on the buttocks, leg, or hand. Striking the child on the face is demeaning as well as dangerous. Slapping is inappropriate at any age. Third, one strike is hard enough to change behavior. Striking the child more than once is more to relieve the parent's anger than to teach the child anything additional. Fourth, striking is

Table 2-3 Characteristics of abusive parents and caretakers with risk degree

Parenting Characteristics	Normal	Moderate risk	Severe risk
Parent beaten or deprived as child	Received empathic "parenting"	Frequent spankings, some bruises; received intermittent "parenting"	Severe beatings; repeated foster homes; no helpful parent model in childhood
Parent has criminal or mental illness record	Not present	Present in part, but rehabilitated for more than five years	Within past five years: prison, psychiatric ward, psychosis, substance addiction or suicide attempt
Parent suspected of abuse in the past	Not present	Official report of mild abuse; children not placed in foster care	Official report of serious abuse; children placed in foster care or died
Parent with poor self-esteem, coping skills and lifelines	Good self-esteem, resilient coping skills, reliable lifelines	Poor self-esteem with stress; intermittent coping skills, few lifelines (usually unreliable)	Chronically poor self-esteem, poor coping skills, no lifelines
Multiple crises or stresses	Not present	Moderate environmental and/or marital problems	Chaotic life-style; severe environmental and/or marital problems
Parent with violent temper outbursts	Not present	Damages property	Attack people
Unrealistic expectations of child's behavior	Not present	Afraid of spoiling child, unrealistic expectations	Intolerance of normal behavior; very strict and rigid parent
Harsh punishment of child	Not present	Current frequent spankings or use of belt, not in head area	Physical punishment of baby prior to crawling; sadistic and/or dangerous punishment
Child difficult and/or provocative (or perceived as such)	Not present	Risk factors present but bonding adequate	Risk factors present and bonding poor

inappropriate before a child has learned to walk. Fifth, physical punishment should not be administered more than three times per day, lest it become a way of life for the child. Sixth, physical punishment should not be used for aggressive misbehavior such as biting or hitting. Physical punishment under such circumstances teaches the child that it is acceptable for a bigger person to strike a smaller person. Aggressive children need to be taught restraint and self-control. Seventh, the danger of causing subdural hematomas by vigorously shaking a young infant should be discussed with the parents or caretakers.

Although striking children with a belt or strap is opposed, keep in mind that this form of punishment is accepted in some ethnic groups. However, these families make it perfectly clear that leaving bruises is unacceptable, as is using a belt on children less than two years old or on any site other than the buttocks or lateral thighs. Clearly, tolerance in this area must remain with strong opposition to harsh discipline. Whenever discussing discipline with a family, one should strive to convince them that they should use alternatives to physical discipline such as a time-out room, time-out chair, verbal disapproval, and removing privileges.

Sexual Abuse

Sexual abuse can be defined as any sexual activity with a child under age 18 by a family-related adult. This may include molestation (fondling or masturbation), intercourse (vaginal, anal, or oral intercourse on a nonassaultive basis), or family-related rape. Sexual abuse is probably the most underdiagnosed type of child abuse and has been called the ''last frontier'' in child abuse. In most cases (90%), the victimized child is a girl. Half the victims are under age 12. The offender is almost always a male (99%). In general, the families are close-knit and secretive, and keep to themselves. Vulvitis, vaginitis, vaginal bleeding, or venereal disease in the prepubertal child must make the physician suspicious of sexual abuse. More than half of these cases provide no positive physical findings or laboratory results, and the child's explicit history of what happened to her must be taken seriously.

Failure to Thrive Due to Nutritional Neglect

Failure to thrive can be defined as an underweight, malnourished condition. A failure-to-thrive child usually has a weight that is below the third percentile and a height and head circumference that are above the third percentile on the growth curves. On physical examination the infants have gaunt faces, prominent ribs, wasted buttocks, and spindly extremities. Failure to thrive is mainly seen in the first two years of life because this is the time of rapid growth as well as dependency on adults for feeding. The causes of failure to thrive are estimated as 30 percent organic, 20 percent underfeeding due to understandable error, and 50 percent underfeeding from parental neglect. The mother may neglect to feed her baby because she feels overwhelmed with responsibilities or is chronically depressed and hostile toward the baby.

A nutritional rehabilitation program is the starting point for reaching a definitive diagnosis in infants with failure to thrive. The child should be hospitalized and placed on unlimited feedings of a regular diet for age. The underweight infant who gains rapidly and easily in the hospital is a victim of underfeeding at home. A rapid weight gain can be defined as more than 1.5 ounces per day sustained for two weeks. A gain of more than 2.0 ounces per day in a one-week period is also diagnostic. Many of these infants also show signs of emotional neglect (such as absence of eye contact or a cuddling response) and need a stimulation program.

Intentional Drugging or Poisoning

Intentional drugging of children involves the administration of a nonprescription or prescription drug that is harmful and not intended for children by parents or caretakers. Sedatives are commonly used. Administering hallucinogenic agents or other recreational drugs to children enhances drug addiction in young children. Intentional poisoning is an uncommon form of child abuse that is often lethal.

Health Care Neglect

When a child with a treatable chronic disease has serious deterioration in such condition because the parents or caretakers repeatedly ignore health care recommendations, health care neglect occurs. Health care neglect may occur in situations where an emergency exists and the parents or caretakers will not acknowledge it as such. Refusals because of religious beliefs, not ignorance, often lead to health care neglect. The child's right, however, to life and health must override the parents' or caretakers' constitutional right to religious freedom. If the disease is incurable, the parents' or caretakers' wishes regarding nonintervention, be they on religious or philosophical grounds, are often respected. Dental neglect must be considered part of the spectrum of health care neglect.

Safety Neglect

Although most accidents are due to a breach in safety and theoretically could have been prevented, the interruption of the fateful event would have required unusual prediction and timing on the part of the parent or caretaker. These are legitimate accidents, and every child has some.

Safety neglect, however, has occurred when injury results from gross lack of supervision. These situations usually involve children less than four years of age, when it is important that parents or caretakers directly supervise them. Too often burns, poisonings, falls, and other preventable accidents occur in children because they were not being watched. Beyond age four most children have a certain degree of freedom, but gross lack of indirect supervision can cause them to become victims of preventable accidents.

Emotional Abuse and Neglect

Emotional abuse can be defined as the continual scapegoating and rejection of a child by parents or caretakers. Severe verbal abuse and berating is often part of emotional abuse. Emotional abuse is often difficult to detect. Psychological terrorism can occur in some cases and presents little difficulty in recognition. Less vivid cases of emotional abuse require the following criteria: (*a*) severe psychopathology and disturbed behavior in the child, of a degree making it unlikely that he/she will be able to function and cope as an adult, documented by a psychiatrist or psychologist; (*b*) abnormal child-rearing practices of the parent or caretaker that have caused a large part of the child's behavior disturbances; and (*c*) the continued refusal by the parent of treatment for the child and himself/herself. These cases can easily be presented as depriving a child of needed mental health care. Situations can be presented with less evidence, however, when the parent or caretaker is floridly psychotic, and hence inadequate to care for the child, or severely depressed, and hence a danger to the child.

Physical Neglect

Some have defined physical neglect as a failure to care for children according to accepted or appropriate standards. It is easy to confuse neglect with poverty, ignorance, or overwhelming problems because it includes things like dirty hair, dirty or inadequate clothing, inadequate lunches, incomplete immunizations, unsanitary home environments, unstimulating environments, inadequate after-school supervision, and excessive work.

Children with physical neglect should be evaluated for coexistent physical abuse. They should also be evaluated for the presence or absence of serious emotional disturbances. In cases of flagrant physical neglect, the parents or caretakers are often very depressed and withdrawn.

Summary

These eight types of child abuse and neglect are clearly injurious to the physical and emotional well-being of children. Although these definitions vary from one state statute to another—or, within state, from one courtroom to another—they should not. When they do, they reflect the failings of a community to protect its children, rather than the lack of uniformity of laws.

Chapter 3

Clinical Diagnosis of Physical Abuse

Barton D. Schmitt

Introduction

Physical abuse or nonaccidental trauma is one of the most common types of child abuse. The yearly incidence in the United States of injuries inflicted by parents or caretakers is generally 700 new cases per million (CDSS, 1977). At least 2,000 children die each year from physical abuse. Approximately 10 percent of children less than five years of age seen by emergency room physicians for trauma have injuries that were inflicted (Holter et al., 1968). A review of the diagnostic acumen necessary for the recognition of inflicted injuries is of paramount importance.

Histories Given for Inflicted Injuries

Although many child abuse diagnoses can be based on physical findings alone, the history of how the injury occurred becomes helpful when a child presents with multiple, nondescript injuries. The following histories are diagnostic or extremely suspicious for nonaccidental trauma (Table 3-1).

Table 3-1 Histories offered for inflicted injuries

Eyewitness history	Unexplained injury	Implausible history
Alleged self-inflicted injury	Alleged sibling-inflicted injury	
Delay in seeking medical care		

Eyewitness History

When a child readily states that a particular parent or caretaker injured him, the history is likely true. When one parent or caretaker accuses the other of injuring a child, the story is usually accurate, if the parents are not engaged in a custody dispute. Partial confessions by a parent or caretaker are not uncommon and are as diagnostic as complete confessions. A parent or caretaker may admit causing one of the injuries but not the others, or may state that intentions of injury were present but action on these impulses did not occur.

Unexplained Injury

Some parents or caretakers deny knowing that their child had any of the injuries discovered. Other parents or caretakers have noticed the physical findings but can offer no explanation as to how the injury happened. These parents would like to have believed that the injury was spontaneous. When pressed, they may become evasive or offer a vague explanation. These explanations are self-incriminating. Most nonabusive parents know exactly how, where, and when their child was hurt. They also show a complete willingness to discuss the accident in detail. In these unexplained injuries, the exact perpetrator can often be identified by learning who was alone with the child when the discomfort and crying commenced.

Implausible History

Many parents offer an explanation for the injury, but one which is implausible and inconsistent with common sense and medical judgment. If the parents offer a blatantly phony history, diagnosis is rather easy. Occasionally, a minor accident is described, yet the injuries are major (e.g., a child reportedly has fallen on to a thick carpet, but has multiple body bruises). Occasionally, the behavior described as leading to the accident is impossible for the child's level of development (e.g., a 10-month-old child who allegedly climbed into a tub and turned on scalding water). Some parents or caretakers make their history implausible by repeatedly changing it.

Alleged Self-Inflicted Injury

An alleged self-inflicted injury in a small baby is most serious. These children can be seriously reinjured or killed if the correct diagnosis is not established. In general, the child who cannot crawl cannot cause a self-inflicted accident. Fractures under this age are almost universally inflicted. Absurd stories should be considered highly unlikely and acted upon accordingly. Histories implying that the child is masochistic should always raise questions (e.g., the child who hurts himself badly during a temper tantrum, gets subdural hematomas by hitting himself with a bottle, climbs up onto a hot radiator, or burns himself up to the elbows by immersing his arm in hot water). Children rarely inflict deliberate injury upon themselves.

Alleged Sibling-Inflicted Injury

When parents or caretakers have difficulty coming up with an explanation, they commonly project the blame onto sibling activity. They may state that the sibling dropped a toy on the injured child or threw a bottle at him. The number and seriousness of the injuries usually contradict this explanation. Only a small percentage of child abuse cases involve siblings.

Delay in Seeking Medical Care

Most nonabusive parents seek immediate care when their child is injured. In contrast, some abused children are not presented for care for a considerable length of time, even when there is a major injury. In the extreme, some are not presented until the child is near death. Approximately one-third of abused children in one study were not presented for care until the morning after the injury. Another one-third came in one to four days after the injury (Smyth, 1972). In these situations, parents or caretakers are usually hoping that the event never occurred, or that the injury will not require medical care. Commonly in the abusive situation, the adult who was with the child at the time of the injury does not come to the health care facility with the child.

Inflicted Bruises

Inflicted bruises occur at typical sites and/or fit recognizable patterns (e.g., human hand marks, human bite marks, strap marks, or bizarre shapes).

Typical Sites

Inflicted bruises are so common at certain body sites that discovering them there is pathognomonic (Table 3-2). Bruises that predominate on the buttocks, lower back, and lateral thighs are almost always related to punishment (i.e., paddling). Likewise, genital or inner-thigh bruises are usually inflicted for toileting mishaps. Injuries to the penis may include pinch marks, cuts, abrasions, a deep groove from having it tied off with a rubber band, or amputation (Slosberg et al., 1978). Injuries to the genital area should also raise the question of sexual abuse, especially when found in girls.

Table 3-2 Typical sites for inflicted bruises

Buttocks and lower back (paddling)	Genitals and inner thighs
Cheek (slap marks)	Earlobe (pinch marks)
Upper lip and frenum (forced feeding)	Neck (choke marks)

Bruises on the cheek are usually secondary to being slapped. Accidental falls rarely cause bruises to the soft tissues of the cheek, but instead involve the skin overlying bony prominences such as the forehead or cheekbone. The outlines of fingers can be evident within the bruise. Bruises on the earlobe are usually due to being pinched. Children who are pinched or pulled by the earlobe usually have a matching bruise on each surface. A child occasionally will suffer a ruptured eardrum from a blow to the ear. Bruises of the upper lip, labial frenum, and floor of the mouth in a child too young to sit up by himself and inadvertently fall forward are usually caused by impatient, forced feedings or by forcing a pacifier or bottle into the child's mouth. Bruises inside the vestibule may remain hidden unless the lip is carefully everted. A history of inconsolable crying often can be obtained in these cases.

Bruises or cuts on the neck are almost always due to being choked or strangled by a human hand, cord, dog collar, or other such instrument. Accidents to this site are extremely rare and should be looked upon with suspicion. Choke marks may be attributed to a resuscitation attempt when in truth they are due to lifting a child off the ground by the neck while slapping him in the face or battering him against a wall. Resuscitative attempts do not leave bruises on the face or neck.

Human Hand Marks

The human hand can leave various types of pressure bruises (Table 3-3). The most common types are grab marks or squeeze marks, oval-shaped bruises that resemble fingerprints. Grab marks are usually due to being forcibly held during violent shaking. The most common site is the forearm. Grab marks of the lower extremities are also common until the child learns to walk. Grab-mark bruises can occur on the cheeks if an adult squeezes a child's face in an attempt to get food or medicine into his mouth. This action leaves a thumb mark bruise on one cheek and two to four finger-mark bruises on the other cheek. Encirclement bruises occur when a child is grabbed about the chest or abdomen. This pattern, when complete, contains as many as eight finger-mark bruises on one side of the body, and two thumb bruises on the other side. The examiner's fingers can fit easily into the configuration.

Table 3-3 Human hand marks

Grab marks or finger-tip bruises	Trunk-encirclement bruises
Linear marks or finger-edge bruises	Slap marks
Hand prints	Pinch marks

Linear grab marks are caused by pressure from the entire finger. The outline or the entire hand print is sometimes seen on the back or at other sites. The hand leaves outline bruises when capillaries at the edge of the injury are stretched enough to rupture. In slap marks to the cheek, two or three parallel linear bruises at finger-width spacing will be seen to run through a more diffuse bruise. The hand can also leave pinch marks, two crescent-shaped bruises facing each other. The shape of the pinch-mark bruise is primarily due to the fingernails.

Human Bite Marks

Human bite marks leave distinctive, often paired, crescent-shaped bruises that contain individual teeth marks. Sometimes the two crescents meet to form a complete ring of bruising. The most common dilemma facing the health care practitioner is to determine if a single bite mark on a child is from a playmate or sibling or from the parents or caretakers. The cusp-to-cusp distance between the maxillary cuspids should be measured. If the distance is greater than three centimeters, the child was probably bitten by an adult or adolescent with a permanent dentition. If the distance is less than three centimeters, the child was probably bitten by another young child with a primary dentition (L. J. Levine, personal communication). In serious injuries with several suspects, the exact perpetrator can often be determined by making an impression of each suspect's dentition and comparing the study casts made from those with photographs or study casts of the bite mark (Levine, 1973).

Strap Marks

Strap marks are one- to two-inch-wide rectangular bruises of various lengths, sometimes covering a curved body surface. These are often caused by a belt. Sometimes the eyelets or buckle of the belt can be discerned. Lash marks are narrow, straight-edged bruises or scratches caused by a thrashing with a tree branch or switch. Loop marks are secondary to being struck with a doubled-over lamp cord, rope, or fan belt. The distal end of the loop strikes with the most force, commonly breaking the skin and leaving loop-shaped scars (Sussman, 1968).

Bizarre Marks

Bizarre-shaped bruises are nearly always inflicted. When a blunt instrument is used in punishment, the resulting bruise or welt will resemble it in shape. Tattooing inflicted with a sharp instrument such as a pin or razor and numerous puncture wounds may be encountered. Circumferential tie marks on the ankles or wrists can be caused when a child is restrained. If a narrow rope or cord is used, the child will be left with circumferential cuts. If a strap or piece of sheeting is used to restrain a child about the wrists or ankles, a friction burn or rope burn may result, usually presenting as a large blister that encircles the extremity. Rope burns have also been seen about the thighs from tying the child to a potty seat. Gag marks may be seen as abrasions that appear near the corner of the mouth. Children may be gagged because of too much screaming or yelling.

Accidental Bruises

A thorough knowledge of common and unusual accidental bruising will help in recognizing inflicted injuries. Understanding unusual customs or practices that leave bruises is also helpful. Lastly, it is important to remember that all bluish discolorations of the skin are not bruises.

Most children periodically acquire one or two bruises during falls or rough activity. The most common site for multiple, easily explained bruises in children of all ages is on the knee and lower leg. These bruises are due to normal falling or bumping into objects while running. Bruises on the forehead are frequent at age two when the child is accomplishing climbing skills.

While bruises from falling usually are circular or nondescript, so are grab marks, ring marks, or blows with a fist. Accidental bruises, however, usually occur on the skin overlying bony prominences (e.g., chin, elbow, forehead, spinous process, greater trochanter, etc.). Nondescript bruises become suspicious as abuse when they occur on the soft parts of the body (e.g., cheek, fleshy part of the arm, buttocks, abdominal wall, etc.). Most falls give one bruise on a single surface. Bruises on multiple body planes are usually inflicted unless there is a history of a tumbling accident. True tumbling accidents also give bruises and abrasions over bony prominences.

Falling down stairs is often offered as an explanation for suspicious bruises on a child. The child who tumbles down the stairs ends up with very few bruises. Therefore, the number and locations of the bruises can speak to an inflicted injury. Babies in the first few months of life commonly scratch themselves on the cheek, ear, nose, or even conjunctiva. This problem is due to long fingernails and disappears if the parent cuts them regularly.

Unusual Bruises

Some common ethnic practices can result in bruises that should not be confused with child abuse. The Vietnamese can induce symmetrical, linear bruises from coin-rubbing (Cao Gio). For symptoms of fever, chills or headaches, the back and chest are covered with hot oil and then massaged in downward strokes with the edge of a coin (Yeatman et al., 1976).

Some teenagers cause multiple petechiae on their chins by sucking on a cup until they create a vacuum and then sliding the cup onto their chin (Lovejoy et al., 1971). Tourniquets can also cause petechiae, especially in children who already have an erythematous rash.

A passionate and prolonged kiss can lead to an area of purpura on the skin. Vigorous sucking on hard candy can leave an area of purpura on the soft palate. Purpura at this site has also been reported with fellatio. Multiple petechiae of the face and neck can occur following vigorous crying, retching, or coughing, due to a sudden increase in superior vena cava pressure. Petechiae and purpura have even been seen in the conjunctiva or mouth as the result of this mechanism.

Pseudobruises

Some skin conditions may be mistaken for bruises. The most common is the Mongolian spot. This birth mark occurs in 95 percent of Blacks, 81 percent of Orientals and American Indians, 70 percent of Chicanos, and 10 percent of Caucasians (Jacobs and Walton, 1976). Lasting from two to three years, they are grayish-blue, do not change color, and have clear-cut margins. Although they commonly occur on the buttocks and back, they can be found anywhere.

Maculae cerulae are unexplained bluish spots on the skin that occur concomitantly with pubic lice and resolve when the lice are treated. Allergic periorbital discoloration is due to long-standing venous congestion from allergic rhinitis and eye allergies. These pseudobruises are usually more brownish than blue, and the discoloration is mainly seen on the lower medial eyelid. The presence of allergies and the duration of the finding points to the correct diagnosis. Hemophilus influenzae can give a bluish cellulitis of the cheek. Afflicted children are sick, run fevers, and their cheek areas are quite tender to palpation.

Inflicted Burns

Approximately 10 percent of physical abuse cases involve burns. Burns from hot solid objects are the easiest to diagnose. These are usually second-degree, without blister formation, and usually involve only one surface of the body. The shape of the burn often resembles its agent and is pathognomonic for child abuse. Abused children are often held against a heating grate or electric hot plate. Cigarette burns give circular, punched-out lesions of uniform size and are often found on the hands or feet. Bullous impetigo should be considered in a differential of burns of this nature.

Hot water burns, normally indicated by blistering, are the most common inflicted burns. Immersion burns occur when a parent holds the thighs against the abdomen and places the buttocks and perineum in scalding liquid as punishment for enuresis or resistance to toilet training. This results in a circular type of burn restricted to the buttocks. With deeper, forced immersions, the burn extends to a level on the thighs and waist. The hands and feet are spared, which is incompatible with falling into a tub or turning the hot water on while in the bathtub. Forcible immersion of a hand or foot as punishment can be suspected when a burn extends well above the wrist or ankle. Toxic epidermal necrolysis should be considered in a differential of scalding burns.

Inflicted Bone Injuries

When physical abuse is suspected in a child less than five years of age, a radiologic bone survey consisting of films of skull, thorax, and long bones should be accomplished. Pelvis and spine films can be accomplished if any of the preceding films are positive. These films are of great diagnostic value, since the clinical findings of fracture often disappear in six or seven days even without orthopedic care. For children over the age of five, radiographs should be obtained only if there is bone tenderness or a limited range of motion on physical examination. If radiographs of a tender site are initially negative, they should be repeated in two weeks to detect any calcification of subperiosteal bleeding or nondisplaced epiphyseal separations that may have occurred. Bone trauma is found in 10 to 20 percent of physically abused children.

Most inflicted fractures are due to wrenching or pulling injuries that damage the metaphysis. The classic early finding is a chip fracture where a corner of the metaphysis of a long bone is torn off, along with the epiphysis and periosteum. From 10 to 14 days later, calcification of the subperiosteal bleeding becomes visible at the periphery. Within four to six weeks after the injury, the subperiosteal calcification will be solid and start to smooth out and remodel. Inflicted fractures of the shaft are usually spiral rather than transverse. Spiral fractures of the femur of a preambulant child are usually inflicted. The most diagnostic radiograph shows injuries to multiple bones at different stages of healing. Such findings imply repeated assaults.

Inflicted Eye Injuries

Ocular damage in the battered child syndrome includes acute hyphema, dislocated lens, traumatic cataract, and detached retina (Mushin, 1971). More than half of these result in permanent impairment of vision affecting one or both eyes. Retinal hemorrhages are also indicative of subdural hematomas in children with unexplained central nervous system findings. Retinal hemorrhage can also occur without clinically important intracranial hemorrhage in children with sudden compression of their chests. This finding is called Purtscher retinopathy (Tomasi, 1975). The differential diagnosis of retinal hemorrhages is direct head trauma, shaking injuries, increased intracranial pressure, hypertension, bleeding disorders, and gymnastic twirling on a horizontal bar. Retinal hemorrhages usually last 10 to 14 days.

Inflicted periorbital bruising is more common than serious eye injuries. Children who have been hit about the eyes with an open or closed hand present with massive swelling and bruising of both eyelids. Most periorbital bruises caused by accidents only involve one side. A child can acquire bilateral periorbital bruises from a single accident, or more precisely from striking a single object. Bilateral periorbital bruises can occur from blood infiltrating from a large bruise on the forehead or from a basilar skull fracture, since blood moves with gravity. However, these children have minimal lid swelling and no lid tenderness. In addition, the onset of the periorbital bruise is delayed one or two days from the time of the injury. Therefore, these situations should not be confused with the child who has been struck about the head and eyes.

Inflicted Head Injuries

Inflicted head injuries include subdural hematomas, subarachnoid hemorrhages, scalp bruises, traumatic alopecia, and subgaleal hematomas.

Subdural Hematomas

Subdural hematoma is the most dangerous inflicted injury, often causing serious sequelae or death. These children present with irritability, vomiting, a decreased level of consciousness, breathing difficulty and apneic episodes, a bulging fontanelle, and/or convulsions (Silber and Bell, 1971). The classic case of subdural hematoma is associated with skull fractures. These fractures are secondary to a direct blow from the parent's or caretaker's hand or from being thrown against a wall or door. Numerous other bruises are often present.

Inflicted subdural hematomas can also occur without skull fractures, scalp bruises, or scalp swelling. In fact, more than one-half of the cases have no fractures (Guthkelch, 1971). These findings used to be called spontaneous subdural hematomas, but recent evidence points to a violent, whiplash shaking mechanism (Caffey, 1974). Rapid acceleration and deceleration of the head as it is in motion leads to tearing of the bridging cerebral veins with bleeding into the subdural space, usually bilaterally. This has been documented from experimental studies on animals and by observation of abusive parents or caretakers. Most of these cases occur in babies less than one year old, who are shaken in an attempt to make them stop crying. Additional diagnostic evidence comes from the presence of retinal hemorrhages in these whiplash subdurals. X-rays of the long bones should also be obtained because they will reveal old or new fractures in 25 percent of the cases (Guthkelch, 1971).

Subarachnoid hemorrhages can result from the same mechanism and may be as common as shaking subdural hematomas. The concept of the spontaneous subdural hematoma in young infants must be discarded to prevent further reinjury or death. Likewise, the diagnosis of chronic subdural hematomas secondary to birth trauma must be viewed with skepticism. Subdural hematomas due to birth injury will often produce acute signs and symptoms within 24 to 48 hours after delivery.

Scalp Bruises

Bruises of the scalp can occur with or without underlying skull fractures or brain injuries. These bruises are often difficult to see because they are deep in the scalp or hidden by the child's hair. Scalp bruises should be suspected with the presence of soft tissue swelling, either on palpation or skull films.

Traumatic Alopecia and Subgaleal Hematomas

Hair-pulling can cause loss of hair (traumatic alopecia) in children. Sometimes the hair is not lost entirely but broken at the ends, secondary to stretching at the site prior to breakage. If the hair-pulling event is recent, the scalp may be tender and a few petechiae may be found at the hair roots. Unlike explained hair loss in patches (alopecia arecita), there are no loose hairs at the periphery of the bald area. Unlike hair loss from disease process, there is no inflammation or scaling of the scalp. Violent and sudden lifting of a child by the hair can also cause a subgaleal hematoma, evidenced by a diffuse, boggy swelling of the scalp. The aponeurosis which connects the occipital and frontalis muscles is lifted off the calvarium and the space rapidly fills with blood. This diagnosis is most likely if the child has braids at the site of the hematoma (Hamlin, 1968). Subgaleal hematoma can also be caused by shearing forces, but probably inflicted if unexplained.

Accidental Head Injuries From Falls

Helfer, Slovis, and Black (1977) in their study of 246 young children who accidentally fell from cribs or beds found that in 80 percent there were no physical injuries. Most of the remainder had single bruises or lacerations. Only one percent of the children had skull fractures, and these were single and linear. Another one percent had fractures at other sites, usually the clavicle or humerus. None of the children had subdural hematomas, epidural hematomas, or any serious life-threatening injury.

Inflicted Abdominal Injuries

Intra-abdominal injuries are the second most common cause of death in abused children (Touloukian, 1968). Unlike the contents of the chest, the abdominal organs are not protected. Table 3-4 lists inflicted abdominal injuries in the approximate order of frequency. Most of the injuries are usually caused by a punch or kick that compresses the organ against the anterior spinal column.

Table 3-4 Inflicted abdominal injuries*

Ruptured liver or spleen	Intestinal perforation
Intramural hematoma of duodenum or proximal jejunum	Pancreatic injury
Ruptured blood vessel	Chylous ascites from injured lymphatic system
Kidney or bladder injury	
Foreign bodies (swallowed or percutaneous)	

*Adapted from Schmitt (1980).

The most common physical finding in inflicted abdominal injuries is a ruptured liver or spleen. These children present with blood loss and shock. Inflicted trauma to the abdomen can cause tears or rents in the small or large intestine. These children often present with advanced peritonitis because of a delay in seeking medical care. A radiograph of the abdomen in an upright position will show free air under the diaphragm.

The most unique abdominal injury is an intramural hematoma of the duodenum or proximal jejunum (Gornall et al., 1972). These children present with projectile vomiting, which is bile-stained if the obstruction is distal, and other signs of gastrointestinal obstruction. With supportive management, the hematoma usually resolves without surgery. Arteries or veins can also be torn in the abdomen, which causes the child to go into shock.

Trauma is the most common cause of acute pancreatitis in children. An anterior blow to the abdomen compresses the pancreas against the vertebral column, and the pancreas can be transected. Children with acute traumatic pancreatitis have symptoms of abdominal tenderness, vomiting, and fever, and their serum and urine amylase levels are markedly elevated. If the initial injury heals, it may progress to a pseudocyst of the pancreas (Penna and Medovy, 1973). These children have persistent abdominal pain and vomiting. Diagnosis is confirmed with the discovery of an abdominal mass on physical examination and the presence on a lateral abdominal radiograph of a soft tissue mass displacing the stomach anteriorally.

Kidney injuries usually result from blows to the back and present with gross hematuria. The bladder may be ruptured by a blow to the lower abdomen. Two unusual cases of child abuse have been reported with chylous ascites and a needle perforation of the liver (Boysen, 1975; Stone et al., 1976).

In all of these conditions, trauma to the abdomen is usually denied (O'Neill et al., 1973). Bruises of the abdominal wall, when present, help to establish the correct diagnosis. Unfortunately, there are no visible bruises or marks on the abdominal wall in more than half of these cases. The abdominal wall is usually relaxed at the time of the injury, and the energy from the blow is mainly absorbed by the internal organs. Child abuse must be suspected in any abdominal crisis of undetermined etiology.

References

Boysen, B. E.: Chylous Ascites. Am. J. Dis. Child. 129:1338, 1975.

Caffey, J.: The Whiplash Shaken Infant Syndrome. Pediatrics 54:396, 1974.

Colorado Department of Social Services (CDSS): Central Registry for Child Protection Report. Denver: CDSS, 1977.

Gornall, P.; Ahmed, S.; Jolleys, A.; et al.: Intra-Abdominal Injuries In the Battered Baby Syndrome. Arch. Dis. Child. 47:211, 1972.

Guthkelch, A. N.: Infantile Subdural Hematoma and Its Relationship to Whiplash Injuries. Brit. Med. J. 2:430, 1971.

Hamlin, H.: Subgaleal Hematoma Caused by Hair-Pull. J. Am. Med. Assoc. 204:339, 1968.

Helfer, R. E.; Slovis, T. L.; and Black, M.: Injuries Resulting When Small Children Fall Out of Bed. Pediatrics 60:633–635, 1977.

Holter, J. C. and Friedman, S. B.: Child Abuse. Early Case Finding in the Emergency Department. Pediatrics 42:128, 1968.

Jacobs, A. H. and Walton, R. G.: Incidence of Birthmarks in the Neonate. Pediatrics 58:218, 1976.

Levine, L. J.: The Solution of a Battered-Child Homocide By Dental Evidence: Report of Case. J. Am. Dent. Assoc. 87:1234, 1973.

Lovejoy, F. H.; Marcuse, E. K.; and Landrigan, P. J.: Two Examples of Purpura Factitia. Clin. Pediat. 11:183, 1971.

Mushin, A. S.: Ocular Damage in the Battered-Baby Syndrome. Brit. Med. J. 3:402, 1971.

O'Neill, J. A.; Meacham, W. F.; Griffin, J. P.; et al.: Patterns of Injury in the Battered Child Syndrome. J. Trauma 13:332, 1973.

Penna, S. D. J. and Medovy, H.: Child Abuse and Traumatic Pseudocyst of the Pancreas. J. Pediat. 83:1026, 1973.

Silber, D. L. and Bell W. E.: The Neurologist and the Physically Abused Child. Neurology 21:991, 1971.

Slosberg, E. J.; Ludwig, S.; Duckett, J.; and Mauro, A. E.: Penile Trauma as a Sign of Child Abuse. Am. J. Dis. Child. 132:719, 1978.

Smyth, S. M.: Child Abuse Syndrome. Brit. Med. J. 3:113, 1972.

Stone, R. K.; Harowitz, A.; San Filippo, J. A.; and Gromisch, D. S.: Needle Perforation of the Liver in an Abused Child. Clin. Pediatr. 15:958, 1976.

Schmitt, B. D.: The Child With Nonaccidental Trauma. In Kempe, C. H. and Helfer, R. E. (ed.) The Battered Child. Chicago: University of Chicago Press, 1980, pp. 128–146.
Sussman, S. J.: Skin Manifestations of the Battered Child Syndrome. J. Pediat. 72:99, 1968.
Tomasi, L. G.: Purtscher Retinopathy in the Battered Child Syndrome. Am. J. Dis. Child 129:1335, 1975.
Touloukian, R. J.: Abdominal Visceral Injuries in Battered Children. Pediatrics 42:642, 1968.
Yeatman, G. W.; Shaw, C.; Barlow, M. J.; and Bartlett, G.: Pseudobattering in Vietnamese Children. Pediatrics 58:616, 1976.

Chapter 4

Oral Facial Injuries in Physical Abuse

Roger G. Sanger

Introduction

Craniofacial trauma with resultant physical injury occurs in more than half of the reported cases of child abuse (Cameron et al., 1966; Skinner and Castle, 1969; Tate, 1971; Becker et al., 1978). It appears likely, then, that dentists frequently treat children who may be victims of physical child abuse. Identification of oral facial injuries per se should present little difficulty to the astute dental clinician. However, ascertainment of suspected child abuse from oral facial injuries can be extremely problematic.

Injuries to the Craniofacial Complex

Physical injuries to the craniofacial complex in child abuse include facial, head, and intraoral injuries in decreasing frequency of occurrence (Becker et al., 1978). Facial injuries include, in order of decreasing frequency: contusions and ecchymoses (bruises), abrasions and lacerations, burns, bone fractures, and bite injuries. Head injuries include skull fracture, subdural hematoma, contusions and ecchymoses (bruises), abrasions and lacerations, and miscellaneous injuries in decreasing frequency. Intraoral injuries include contusions and ecchymoses (bruises), abrasions and lacerations, and trauma to the dentition in decreasing frequency (Becker et al., 1978).

These physical injuries then, because of their high incidence in reported cases of physical child abuse, must be evaluated by the clinician with a high degree of suspicion for child abuse. Type and location of physical injury should prompt the clinician to further investigate the circumstances to determine if other indicators of physical abuse are present. The oral cavity is often the central focus for physical abuse because of its significance in communication and nutrition.

Indicators of Abuse to the Oral Facial Complex

Suspicious physical injuries of the oral facial complex are often present as pattern injuries where the injury represents or patterns the object responsible for the actual tissue damage. Patterning combined with the type and location of the injury are usually observable indicators of physical abuse. The following will delineate certain observable indicators by location, type, and pattern of injury.

Bruises
- On the face indicating slapping by fingers and hand
- On the face indicating grabbing by fingers and hand
- On the face resembling an instrument
- Around the neck indicating restraint
- To the perioral structures indicating gagging
- On the face indicating bite marks
- In the oral cavity, especially the palate, vestibules, and floor of the mouth indicating blunt trauma from blunt instrument or finger

Lacerations
- Detached labial or lingual frenum indicating blunt trauma from instrument or finger
- Lacerations and puncture wounds on the face or in the oral cavity resembling an instrument

Burns
- Of the face, resembling an instrument
- Of the oral cavity indicating instrument placement
- Resulting from toxic chemicals placed in the oral cavity
- Resulting from scalding liquids placed in the oral cavity

Miscellaneous Injuries
- Ocular trauma indicating blunt trauma or pattern injury by instrument
- Auricular trauma indicating blunt trauma (pugilistic appearance) or pattern injury by instrument
- Tympanic membrane perforations
- Facial fractures indicating blunt trauma or pattern injury from instrument

Injuries to the Dentition
- Traumatized or avulsed teeth indicating blunt trauma or pattern injury from instrument
- Discolored teeth indicating repeated trauma

Besides type, location, and patterning, other indicators of physical abuse to the oral facial complex include multiplicity, resolution, and appropriateness. Injuries may be sustained as the result of single or multiple incidents. Multiplicity or the presence of more than one physical injury can be reason to suspect nonaccidental trauma. Injuries in different stages of healing or resolution are also suspicious as nonaccidental trauma. In addition, injuries may not be appropriate for the age, behavioral maturity, developmental maturity, or physical maturity of the child and should be suspected as nonaccidental trauma. Panoramic and intraoral radiographic surveys are invaluable in the analysis of these six indicators. When any is present, the level of suspicion for physical child abuse increases (Schwartz et al., 1977;

Sopher, 1977; McNeese and Hebeler, 1977; Sognnaes and Blain, 1979; Davis et al., 1979; Kittle et al., 1981).

Self-Inflicted Injuries to the Oral Facial Complex

Self-infliction of injuries to the oral facial complex must be considered when evaluating any oral facial injury. Self-infliction of injury is common in young children for reasons that may include the need for sympathy, the need for attention, and personal gratification (Blanton et al., 1977). Self-infliction of injury is also possible as a manifestation of a mental retardation syndrome, physical disability syndrome, or emotional disorders.

Self-inflicted injuries are again very difficult to diagnose without certain indicators. In general, the injuries of self-inflicted trauma (Blanton et al., 1977):

- Are manifestations of a syndrome and have been documented in the literature
- Do not correspond to a known disease process
- Reveal bizarre configurations
- Reveal unusual groupings and distributions
- Are found in body areas accessible to the teeth and/or fingers
- Are usually multiple and in different stages of healing or resolution

Discrepant History and Circumstances of Injury

Often present with suspicious physical abuse in children is the discrepant or conflicting history and circumstances surrounding the occurrence of the injury. As with other systemic injuries, this discrepancy or conflict is common for oral facial injuries in physical child abuse.

In addition to the inappropriateness of the injury for the age and behavioral, developmental, and physical maturity of the victim, the following should be considered as discrepant or conflicting history and circumstances (ten Bensel and King, 1975):

- Different or conflicting history and circumstances given by one or more persons
- Physical injury and reported circumstances do not match
- Physical injury attributed to nonexistent medical problem or history
- Physical injury attributed to accident-prone child or other child/sibling
- Delay in seeking health care for physical injury
- Repeated occurrences of similar injuries with conflicting histories and circumstances
- Suspicious behavior of adult and/or child
- Abnormal growth and development attributable to past and/or present physical injury

Differential Diagnosis

The dental professional must ascertain to the best of his/her professional ability and in good faith whether the physical injuries of the oral facial complex being evaluated are the result of accident, self-infliction, or nonaccidental second-party assault. Physical abuse is not always an absolute diagnosis, even for the most astute and informed clinician. If reasonable suspicion of nonaccidental injury remains after a thorough differential diagnosis has been performed, the dental professional should establish a tentative diagnosis of physical child abuse and proceed according to professional ethics and legislative mandates. Documentation and collection of physical evidence is of paramount concern but the dental professional must not fail to provide treatment for the physical injuries. Both of these topics are discussed in later chapters.

Summary

The dental professional, when encountering physical injury to the oral facial complex, must accomplish a thorough examination and history appropriate for the injury and document the procedures. Crucial to the decision of suspected child abuse, the dental professional must ascertain if the encountered injuries are the result of accident, self-infliction, or nonaccidental second-party assault. A differential diagnosis of the injuries may be less difficult if the dental professional considers the following indicators collectively rather than separately:

- Type
- Location
- Pattern characteristics
- Multiplicity
- Resolution
- Appropriateness for the child's:
  - age
  - behavioral maturity
  - developmental maturity
  - physical maturity
- History and circumstances surrounding occurrence

References

Becker, D. B.; Needleman, H. L.; and Kotelchuck, M.: Child Abuse and Dentistry: Orofacial Trauma and Its Recognition by Dentists. J. Am. Dent. Assoc. 97:24, 1978.

Blanton, P. L.; Hurt, W. C.; and Largent, M. D.: Oral Factitious Injuries. J. Periodontol. 48:33, 1977.

Cameron, J.; Johnson, H.; and Camps, F.: The Battered Child Syndrome. Med. Sci. Law 6:1, 1966.

Davis, G. R.; Domoto, P. K.; and Levy, R. L.: The Dentist's Role in Child Abuse and Neglect—Issues, Identification and Management. J. Dent. Child. 46:185–192, 1979.

Kittle, P. E.; Richardson, D. S.; and Parker, J. W.: Two Child Abuse/Child Neglect Examinations for the Dentist. J. Dent. Child. 48:175–180, 1981.

McNeese, M. C. and Hebeler, J. R.: The Abused Child—A Clinical Approach to Identification and Management, Clin. Symp. 29(5):1–36, 1977.

Schwartz, S.; Woolridge, E.; and Stege, D.: Oral Manifestations and Legal Aspects of Child Abuse. J. Am. Dent. Assoc. 95:586–591, 1977.
Skinner, A. and Castle, R.: A Retrospective Study. London: National Society for Prevention of Cruelty to Children, 1969, p. 1.
Sognnaes, R. F. and Blain, S. M.: Child Abuse and Neglect, I—Diagnostic Criteria of Special Interest to Dentists. IADR (ABS), 1104, J. Dent. Res. 58:367, 1979.
Sopher, I. M.: The Dentist and the Battered Child Syndrome. Dent. Clin. North Am. 21:113–122, 1977.
Tate, R. J.: Facial Injuries Associated with the Battered Child Syndrome. Br. J. Oral Surg. 9:41, 1971.
ten Bensel, R. W. and King, K.: Neglect and Abuse of Children: Historical Aspects, Identification and Management. J. Dent. Child. 42:348, 1975.

Chapter 5

Oral Facial Lesions in Sexual Abuse

Paul S. Casamassimo

Introduction

Sexual abuse is generally recognized as the most disturbing form of child abuse. Cultural and social taboos against incest and other forms of sexual abuse have led to the belief that sexual abuse of children is rare. To the contrary, recent estimates put the current United States yearly incidence of sexual child abuse at between 60,000 and 100,000 cases (DHEW, 1978). The reluctance of parents and family to report sexual abuse, their fear of social repercussions, their hesitation to subject children to questioning, and professional ignorance and hesitation to investigate sexual abuse may contribute to gross underreporting.

Sexual abuse is defined variably according to individual, medical, and legal interpretations. The National Center on Child Abuse and Neglect considers a child sexually abused when he/she is used by an adult for the sexual stimulation of the perpetrator or a third party. The definition includes such specific acts as fondling, exhibitionism, forcible rape, pornography, incest, and the gamut of sexual acts including oral sexual contact. Complications of sexual abuse are psychological and emotional trauma, pregnancy, venereal disease, and physical trauma (Jaffe et al., 1975). This chapter will concentrate on these last two morbidity factors, while incorporating aspects of psychological and emotional trauma as they relate to epidemiology into a clinical picture of sexual abuse useful to the dental professional.

Identifying Sexual Abuse in Children

Problems for Dental Professionals

The infrequent reporting of sexual abuse by dental professionals is not unexpected, especially in view of a suspected low reporting rate by physicians and other professionals (Rosenfeld, 1979). The current burst of interest in the dental professional's role in identification of child abuse has largely ignored sexual abuse in children. Literature has focused on the battered child, with only an occasional mention of sexual abuse (ten Bensel et al., 1977; Laskin, 1978; Becker et al., 1978).

Other factors contributing to the problem of low identification are (*a*) the dental professional's lack of familiarity with sexual lesions of the oral and perioral regions, (*b*) the variable manifestation of infectious lesions, (*c*) the relatively low occurrence in both pediatric and family dental practice, and (*d*) the dental professional's reluctance to become involved in an area of abuse that he or she may see as outside of their purview. A dental professional does not have the sanction to either perform corroborating physical examination of genitalia or hold private discussions of sexual matters with children in the office setting (Kittle et al., 1981). This limitation may in itself account for underreporting.

General Appraisal

The sexually abused child is identified most frequently without a chief complaint or history quite serendipitously by the acutely observant dental professional. Detection of sexual abuse occurs only with a high incidence of suspicion on the part of any professional (Herjanic and Wilbois, 1978). The first diagnostic procedure performed by the dentist is most often a general appraisal and not a comprehensive history. Historical data tend to solidify the diagnosis of child abuse rather than to provide the practitioner with directions for initial clinical data gathering.

Studies of child sexual abuse suggests trends rather than a characteristic physical picture of the sexually abused child. Children from infancy to late adolescence can be victims of sexual abuse, with the mean age around 10 to 11 years (Jaffe et al., 1975; Tilelli et al., 1980; Luther and Price, 1980). Girls tend to be victimized far more often than boys (Jaffe et al., 1975; Sgroi, 1979; Scherzer and Lala, 1980; Luther and Price, 1980). Boys, however, more often have accompanying physical injury (Ellerstein and Canavan, 1980). Sexual and physical abuse can occur together, with younger children showing signs of physical abuse more often than older ones (Jaffe et al., 1975; Tilelli et al., 1980; Cline, 1980). This association suggests that when physical abuse is suspected, appropriate diagnostic procedures be instituted to identify sexual abuse as well.

Behavioral changes may accompany sexual abuse. These can include psychosomatic problems, seductive behavior toward adults, aggressive behavior, identity conflicts, guilt and ambivalence, and acting out behaviors (Nakashima and Zakus, 1977; Rosenfeld, 1979; Cline, 1980). It is unlikely that the dental professional would immediately associate behavioral change with sexual abuse. However, behavior change in the presence of identifiable lesions or in a child with whom the practitioner has established a sound relationship should encourage further investigation.

Historical Data Gathering

Historical data can help to confirm a suspicion of sexual child abuse. Studies of sexual abuse suggest individual and familial characteristics that may be associated with clinical findings. Perhaps the most common finding is family dysfunction including sexual difficulties between parents, shared fears of family disintegration by all members, a withdrawn and condoning mother, and an ineffectual, nonaggressive, and dependent father (Nakashima and Zakus, 1977; Weitzel et al., 1978; Nakashima and Zakus, 1979; Brown, 1979; Meiselman, 1979). About one-half of the cases reported in one study came from single-parent families (Scherzer and Lala, 1980).

Familial involvement in sexual abuse may be as high as 50 percent, with father/daughter and stepfather/stepdaughter cases most likely, although father/son incest or other homosexual acts are possible (Burgess and Holmstrom, 1975; Cline, 1980). Sexual abuse often occurs in "safe havens" such as the home and is often perpetrated by family or trusted adults (Scherzer and Lala, 1980). The abused child will usually know the assailant, most often male, and may have an abused sibling (Tilelli et al., 1980; Luther and Price, 1980). No standard profile of the perpetrator exists, as sexually abusive parents/adults come from all strata of society including those where families appear stable and well-functioning (Nakashima and Zakus, 1977; Luther and Price, 1980).

The sexually abused child may have a history of recent difficulties with friends, failure in school, isolation from peers, encopresis, or enuresis (Rosenfeld, 1979). Sexually abused children are often repeatedly victimized (Tilelli et al., 1980; Cline, 1980). Children less than eight to 10 years old may recount an episode of sexual abuse without intercourse, while older children are often victims of sexual intercourse (Tilelli et al., 1980).

History-taking for child abuse is difficult in general, but is even more so for the dental professional, especially when sexual abuse is suspected. In contrast to the medical literature, which suggests private interviewing, the dental literature supports questioning in the presence of another adult to preclude medicolegal confrontation (Kittle et al., 1981).

Oral Facial Manifestations

Oral facial manifestations in sexual abuse include lesions of infectious venereal disease and traumatic injuries from oral sexual acts. Venereal lesions of gonorrhea, syphilis, and viral infection are well-documented in children and young adults, with many authors stating that venereal lesions in children are pathognomonic of sexual abuse (Mininberg and Rudick, 1976; Nelson et al., 1976; Low et al., 1977; Folland et al., 1977; Potterat et al., 1978; Seidel et al., 1979).

The appearance of venereal infection in the handicapped and chronically ill child should not be assumed to be opportunistic; these children may be easy prey for sexual abuse because of physical or intellectual disability or because such contact yields needed sexual or emotional gratification (Burgess and Holstrom, 1975).

Gonorrhea

The most commonly identified infectious venereal disease is gonorrhea, which is

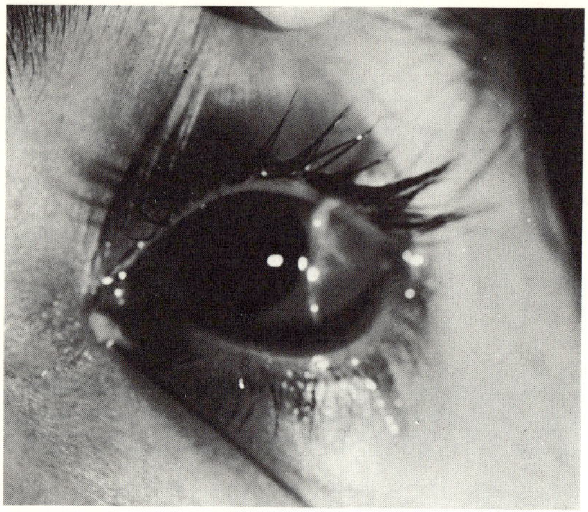

Fig. 5-1 Gonococcal conjunctivitis of the eye demonstrating erythema and vesiculopustular formations. A positive culture for *Neisseria gonorrhoeae* was obtained. The patient also demonstrated positive signs and symptoms of gonococcal pharyngitis.

most often detected after complaints of vaginal or urethral discomfort or signs and symptoms of sore throat or conjunctivitis (Low et al., 1977; Folland et al., 1977; Potterat et al., 1978). Gonococcal infections from sexual abuse are more commonly identified in girls, although they do occur in boys. Estimates of oral infection in those patients who have positive cultures range between 10 and 20 percent (Nelson et al., 1976; Low et al., 1977). Transmission is often through a family member who may or may not be asymptomatic (Potterat et al., 1978).

The oral manifestations of gonorrhea are highly variable and can involve lips, tongue, palate, or pharynx and face with a variety of appearances ranging from mild erythema to frank ulceration and from vesiculopustular to pseudomembranous lesions (Chue, 1975; Merchant and Schuster, 1977) (Fig. 5-1). Although a variety of lesions are possible, pharyngitis appears to be a frequent finding in child sexual abuse (Silber et al., 1977; Silber, 1978). Even pharyngeal signs can vary from mild erythema to frank ulceration and swelling of pharyngeal tissues. Positive cultures are possible in the absence of clinical signs (Low et al., 1977; Silber, 1978). These asymptomatic carriers suggest that the incidence of gonococcal infection from abuse may be much higher than data indicate.

Differential diagnosis in the case of pharyngitis should include acute tonsillitis, pharyngeal streptococcal infection, scarlet fever, or mononucleosis (Jamsky, 1977). A positive culture for *Neisseria gonorrhoeae* confirms the diagnosis. A negative culture for B-hemolytic streptococci or a suspicious history of accompanying genital signs and symptoms should encourage pursuit of possible sexual abuse (Silber et al., 1977; Silber, 1978).

In cases of isolated lesions or a generalized gonococcal stomatitis, various possible etiologies need to be evaluated and excluded (Kohn et al., 1972). Unusual lesions in or around the mouth should arouse suspicion (Herjanic and Wilbois, 1978). Most authorities agree that a confirmed case of gonorrhea in a child assumes sexual transmission (Folland et al., 1977; Potterat et al., 1978). Because of the rare and variable nature of oral gonorrhea, its potential for asymptomatic infection, and its mimicry of other infectious childhood diseases, its identification in routine oral examination is questionable. The most effective treatment is with an injection of aqueous penicillin.

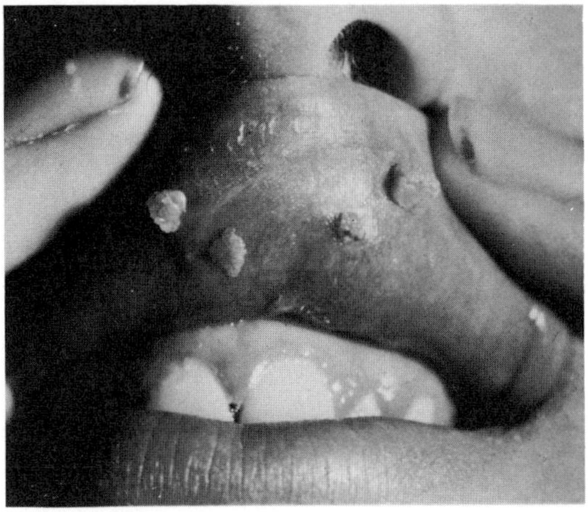

Figs. 5-2 and 5-3 Condyloma acuminatum or venereal wart of the lips. These lesions can be singular or multiple in occurrence and of viral origin.

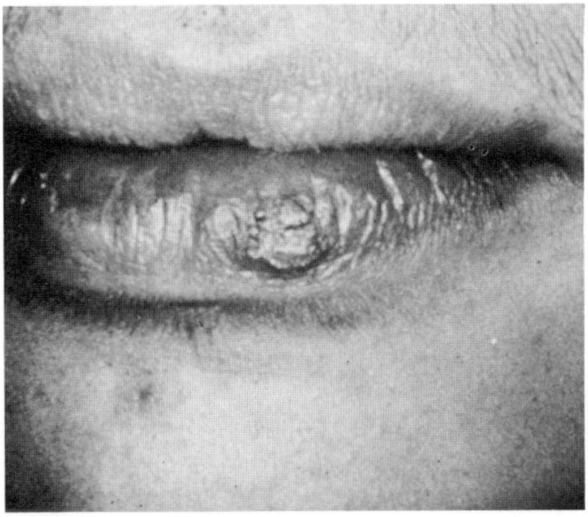

Figure 5-3

Condyloma Acuminatum

Condyloma acuminatum or venereal wart has been identified in children who are suspected of being abused (Mininberg and Rudick, 1976; Seidel et al., 1979) (Figs. 5-2 and 5-3). These raised, pedunculated cauliflower-like lesions can be isolated or multiple in occurrence. They are caused by a virus similar to that causing common skin warts. These lesions occur after repeated sexual contact with a carrier in the oral, anal, or genital region (Fiumara, 1976; Seidel et al., 1979). Unlike gonorrhea, the venereal wart poses no threat of serious injury to health, but is highly suggestive of sexual abuse and should prompt further investigation and documentation by the dentist. Treatment is to stop contact and surgically remove the lesion.

Syphilis

Oral syphilis appears to be a relatively rare finding in child sexual abuse, though

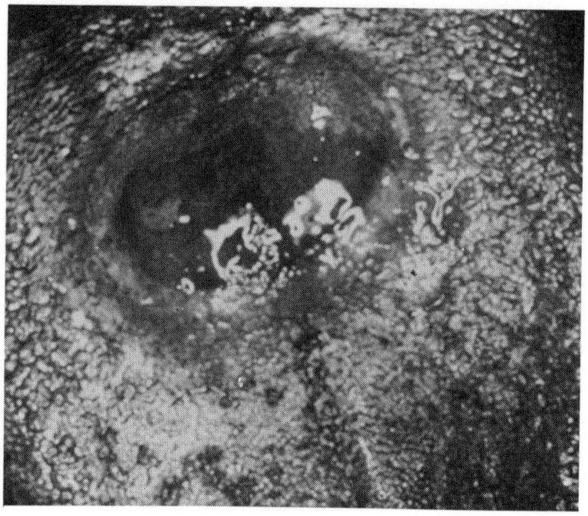

Fig. 5-4 Syphilitic chancre of the tongue demonstrating classical ulceration at the site of inoculation. A positive culture for *Treponema pallidum* was obtained.

occurrence of the disease in children nearly always indicates sexual abuse. Culturing for *Treponema pallidum* is standard protocol in suspected cases (Pascoe, 1979). Syphilis has a 21-day incubation period and manifests on the dermus or lip early as a papule at the site of inoculation ulcerating to form the classic chancre (Fig. 5-4). Primary syphilis can also appear as a red gingival lesion, though this is rare (Alexander, 1975). Secondary syphilis can manifest as a flu-like disorder with regional lymphadenopathy. A mucous patch and split papule and condyloma lata can occur in the oral and perioral region (Fiumara et al., 1978).

Oral syphilis is transmittable through digital contact. Historical investigation may suggest father/son contact or another homosexual contact since syphilis is epidemic in the male homosexual population, yet found in lesser proportions than gonorrhea and other venereal infections in the heterosexual population (Judson, 1977; Holmes and Martin, 1978). Treatment of syphilis is with oral penicillin.

Herpes Progenitalis

Herpes Progenitalis presents still another possible infection in sexual-abuse origin (Fiumara, 1976). The Herpes Type II virus is a rare agent of the oral cavity with most infections confined to the genital area. However, cases of oral infection in conjunction with genital infection have been identified (Needleman, personal communication, 1981). The oral lesions can vary from isolated classical herpetic lesions to viral pharyngitis to an appearance suggestive of primary herpetic gingivostomatitis (Fig. 5-5). Diagnosis is based on identification of the Type II virus. Without a suspicion of child sexual abuse it is unlikely that even the astute diagnostician would suspect oral-genital transmission. Treatment remains palliative and includes minimizing transmission to others.

Erythema/Petechial Palate

Erythema or petechiae of the hard and soft palate associated with fellatio provides

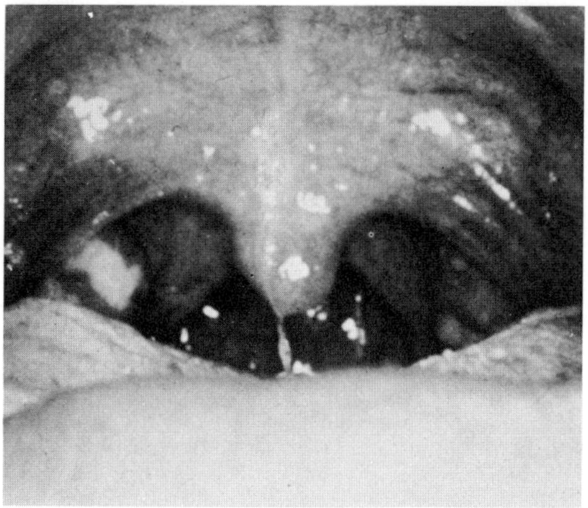

Fig. 5-5 Herpes progenitalis of the tonsillar area demonstrating as tonsilitis and pharyngitis. A positive culture for herpes virus type II was obtained.

the clinician with a simpler differential diagnosis. The lesions may be areas of erythema or single or multiple petechiae, or ecchymotic areas with accompanying erythema located at the junction of the hard and soft palate (Schlesinger et al., 1975; Giansanti et al., 1975). They are painless and regress without treatment once the abusive act is stopped. Systemic diseases such as leukemia, platelet diseases, or mononucleosis can manifest similar signs, but once ruled out leave sexually induced trauma from suction as a prime suspect.

Other Venereal Diseases

It should be noted that oral infections such as moniliasis and trichomonas vaginitis can be transmitted to the oral cavity. These infections, if identified in young children, should prompt the dental professional to rule out abuse (Fiumara, 1976).

Diagnostic Procedures

Collection of specimens for laboratory analysis to verify venereal disease and for use as evidence is of critical importance. Fragility of organisms requires proper sampling techniques, and legal guidelines for evidential admissibility demand specific procedures for collection of specimens.

In the case of suspected gonorrhea, a sterile cotton swab should be used to obtain a sample suitable for culture. If sodomy is suspected, a cotton swab should be used to obtain samples from the pharynx, floor of the mouth, and other recesses of the oral cavity. The swabs are then smeared on slides and air-dried. At least one swab should be preserved in one cubic centimeter of normal saline. Pubic hair should be retrieved from the oral cavity and placed in an envelope labelled with patient name, date, time, and site of sample (Pascoe, 1979).

In cases of other infectious diseases, appropriate culturing should be done to assist in diagnosis and documentation. This may include obtaining an exudate and tissue sample for herpetic infection, or a surface scraping for moniliasis (Daniel, 1977). The child with suspected syphilis should be referred for serologic testing. In all cases of clinically identifiable lesions, photographs and recording of clinical examination findings are paramount.

Summary

Child sexual abuse may have oral manifestations. Identification of sexual abuse may be difficult because it is rare and may occur without signs of physical abuse. In addition, the dental professional has little exposure to oral sexual lesions, which are often variable in appearance. Little has been written in the dental literature to acquaint the dentist with signs of sexual abuse in children, or to provide him/her with methods for gathering data about suspected cases. Child sexual abuse will be overlooked unless accompanied by a positive history and/or clinical evidence of physical abuse, or manifested in a discrete lesion defying alternate diagnosis.

References

Alexander, W. N.: Venereal Disease and the Dentist. J. Academy Gen. Dent. 23(2):14–58, 1975.

Becker, D. B.; Needleman, M. L.; and Kotelchuck, M.: Child Abuse and Dentistry: Orofacial Trauma and its Recognition by Dentists. J. Am. Dent. Assoc. 97:24–28, 1978.

Brown, S.: Clinical Illustrations of the Sexual Misuse of Girls. Child Wel. 58:435–442, 1979.

Burgess, A. W. and Holmstrom, L. L.: Sexual Trauma of Children and Adolescents. Nurs. Clin. North Am. 10:551–563, 1975.

Chue, P. W. Y.: Gonorrhea—Its Natural History, Oral Manifestations, Diagnosis, Treatment and Prevention. J. Am. Dent. Assoc. 90:1297–1301, 1975.

Cline, F.: Dealing with Sexual Abuse in Children. Nurse Pract. 5(3):52–54, 1980.

Daniel, W. A.: Adolescents in Health and Disease. St. Louis: The C.V. Mosby Co., 1977, pp. 166–176.

Department of Health, Education, and Welfare (DHEW): Child Sexual Abuse: Incest, Assault, and Sexual Exploitation. A Special Report from the National Center on Child Abuse and Neglect. DHEW Publ. No. (OHDS) 79-30166, 1978.

Ellerstein, N. S. and Canavan, J. W.: Sexual Abuse of Boys. Am. J. Dis. Child. 134:255–257, 1980.

Fiumara, N. J.: Venereal Diseases of the Oral Cavity. J. Oral Med. 31(2):36–40, 1976.

Fiumara, N. J.; Giunta, J. L.; and Collins, P. S.: Nasolabial Condylomata Lata: Report of Case. Sex. Transm. Dis. 5:112–114, 1978.

Folland, D. S.; Burke, R. E.; Hinman, A. R.; and Schaffner, W.: Gonorrhea in Preadolescent Children: An Inquiry Into Source of Infection and Mode of Transmission. Pediatrics 60:153–156, 1977.

Giansanti, J. G.; Cramer, J. R.; Weathers, D. R.: Palatal Erythema: Another Etiologic Factor. Oral Surg. Oral Med. Oral Pathol. 40(3):379–381, 1975.

Herjanic, B. and Wilbois, R. P.: Sexual Abuse of Children. J. Am. Med. Assoc. 239:301–333, 1978.

Holmes, K. K. and Martin, D.: Sexually Transmitted Diseases/Advances in Management. Postgr. Med. 64(3):121–136, 1978.

Jaffe, A. C.; Dynneson, L.; and ten Bensel, R. W.: Sexual Abuse in Children, An Epidemiologic Study. Am. J. Dis. Child. 129:689–692, 1975.

Jamsky, R. J.: Gonococcal Tonsilitis: Report of a Case. Oral Surg. Oral Med. Oral Pathol. 44(2):197–200, 1977.

Judson, F. N.: Sexually Transmitted Diseases in Gay Men. Sex. Transm. Dis. 4(2):76–78, 1977.

Kittle, P. E.; Richardson, D. S.; and Parker, J. W.: Two Child Abuse/Child Neglect Examinations for the Dentist. J. Dent. Child. 48:175–180, 1981.

Kohn, S. R.; Shaffer, J. F.; and Chomenko, A. G.: Primary Gonococcal Stomatitis. J. Am. Med. Assoc. 219(1):86, 1972.

Laskin, D. M.: The Recognition of Child Abuse. J. Oral Surg. 36(5):349, 1978.
Low, R. C.; Cho, C. T.; and Dudding, B. A.: Gonococcal Infections in Young Children, Studies on the Social, Familial and Clinical Aspects of 11 Instances. Clin. Pediat. 16:623–626, 1977.
Luther, S. L. and Price, J. H.: Child Sexual Abuse: A Review. J. Sch. Health 50(3):161–165, 1980.
Meiselman, K. C.: Incest, a Psychological Study of Causes and Effects with Treatment Recommendations. San Francisco: Jossey-Bass, 1979.
Merchant, H. W. and Schuster, G. S.: Oral Gonococcal Infection. J. Am. Dent. Assoc. 95:807–809, 1977.
Mininberg, D. T. and Rudick, D. H.: Urethral Condyloma Acuminata in Male Children. Pediatrics 57:571–572, 1976.
Nakashima, I. and Zakus, G.: Incest: Review and Clinical Experience. Pediatrics 60:696–701, 1977.
Nakashima, I. and Zakus, G.: Incestuous Families. Pediat. Ann. 8(5):29–42, 1979.
Nelson, J. D.; Mohs, E.; Dajani, A. S.; and Plotkin, S. A.: Gonorrhea in Preschool and School-Aged Children, Report of the Prepubertal Gonorrhea Cooperative Study Group. J. Am. Med. Assoc. 236:1359–1364, 1976.
Pascoe, D. J.: Management of Sexually Abused Children. Pediat. Ann. 8(5):44–58, 1979.
Potterat, J. J.; Markewich, G. S.; and Rothenberg, R.: Prepubertal Infections with Neisseria Gonorrhoeae: Clinical and Epidemiologic Significance. Sex. Trans. Dis. 5(1):1–3, 1978.
Rosenfeld, A. A.: The Clinical Management of Incest and Sexual Abuse of Children. J. Am. Med. Assoc. 242:1761–1764, 1979.
Scherzer, L. N. and Lala, P.: Sexual Offenses Committed Against Children. Clin. Pediat. 19:679–685, 1980.
Schlesinger, S.; Borbotsina, J.; and O'Neill, L.: Petechial Hemorrhages of the Soft Palate Secondary to Fellatio. Oral Surg. Oral Med. Oral Pathol. 40:376–378, 1975.
Seidel, J.; Zonana, J.; and Totten, E.: Condylomata Acuminata as a Sign of Sexual Abuse in Children. J. Pediat. 95:553–554, 1979.
Sgroi, S. M.: Pediatric Gonorrhea Beyond Infancy. Pediat. Ann. 8(5):73–87, 1979.
Silber, T. J.; Controni, G.; and Korin, D. E.: Pharyngeal Gonorrhea in Children and Adolescents. Clin. Proc. Child. Hosp. Natl. Med. Cent. 33(4):79–81, 1977.
Silber, T. J.: Pharyngeal Gonorrhea in Children. Pediatrics 61:674, 1978.
ten Bensel, R. W.; King, K. J.; and Bastien, S. A.: Child Abuse and Neglect: History, Identification and Reporting. Dent. Hyg. 51:119–125, 1977.
Tilelli, J. A.: Turek, D.; and Jaffe, A. C.: Sexual Abuse of Children. New Engl. J. Med. 302:319–323, 1980.
Weitzel, W. D.; Powell, B. J.; and Penick; E. C.: Clinical Management of Father-Daughter Incest. Am. J. Dis. Child. 132(2):127–130, 1978.

Chapter 6

Bite Marks in Child Abuse

Lowell J. Levine

Introduction

Bite marks are found on a significant number of child abuse victims. Every professional who might come into contact with these children must learn to *recognize* this special type of pattern injury, understand the *significance* of it, know how to *document* it, and be able to *refer* the evidence for competent *interpretation*.

Most child abuse cases with bite marks documented in the literature involve homicides or severe assaults because the dentists best trained to recognize the evidence, the forensic odontologists, are traditionally associated with medical examiner, coroner, or law enforcement agencies. Although these cases seem to exhibit a pattern of severe head trauma associated with a finding of bite marks on the victim, this does not preclude the existence of bite marks as the solitary lesions indicative of child abuse.

Recognition

Types

Physically abused children may exhibit healed, healing, and/or fresh bite marks as well as other tissue injury. There may be single or multiple bite marks inflicted during solo or multiple assault episodes. Bite marks on nonabused children may be from a single incident and may exhibit single or multiple, contemporaneous, bite marks.

Descriptions

A bite mark is a patterned injury exhibiting the obvious, gross features of a dentition (see Figs. 6-1–6-8). In the case of a bite mark of human origin involving both dental arches (anterior and premolar teeth) an elliptical or ovoid pattern will be seen. If the characteristic pattern of the maxillary canine teeth can be interpreted, the distance between the two canine marks will measure from 2.5 to 4.5 centimeters. A canine-to-canine distance of less than 3.0 centimeters indicates the

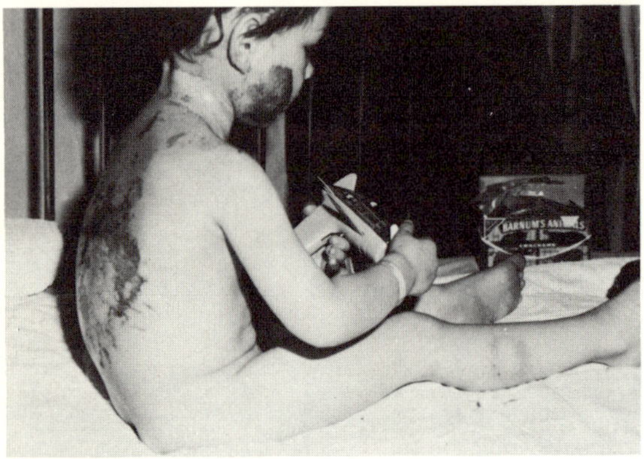

Fig. 6-1 Child with burns of the face, back, and groin, which his guardian claimed occurred when he pulled a pot of boiling water off a stove. Note the adult-size bite mark on the right calf, approximately the same age as the burn injuries.

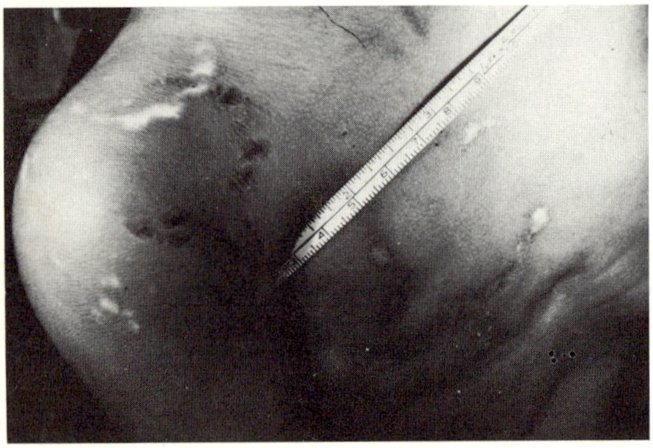

Fig. 6-2 Healed and healing bite marks on a battered child homicide victim.

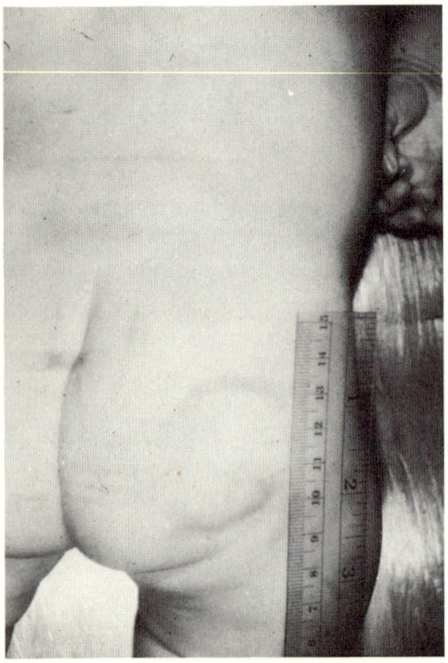

Fig. 6-3 Bite mark on the buttock of a child homicide victim.

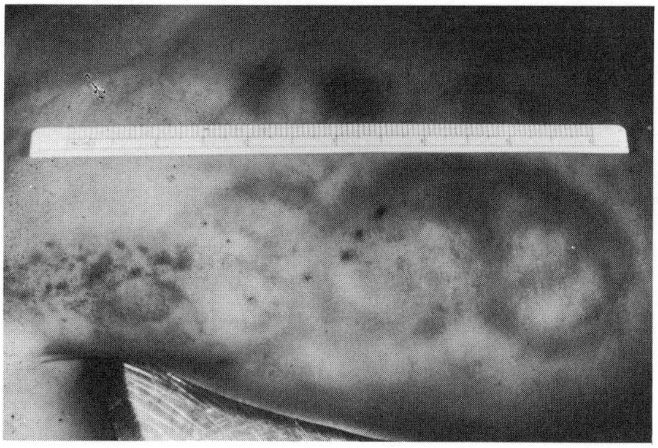

Fig. 6-4 Multiple bite marks on an infant homicide victim.

bite mark may have been caused by the deciduous dentition of a child. Partial marks are interpreted by attempting to determine overall size.

Class characteristics of teeth categories are reflections of the shapes of their incisal or occlusal areas. Incisors cause rectangles or portions of rectangles. Canines cause triangles or portions of triangles, usually with the "apex" towards the facial. Premolars or bicuspids cause triangles, circles, or diamonds. The rectangular marks left by maxillary and mandibular incisors reflect differences in their mesiodistal widths. Perforations rather than whole rectangular shapes may sometimes be noted in the incisor areas, and are caused by the incisal angle-interproximal relationship.

The portion of the bite mark caused by maxillary arch is sometimes more diffuse, and by the mandibular more distinct. This is caused by the dynamics of biting. The maxilla is fixed to the skull and is used for holding, while the mandible is movable and used for cutting. Skin slippage causes the more diffused appearance of the maxillary characteristics in certain cases.

Locations

Bite marks have been found on child abuse victims everywhere on the body, including the genitalia. The bite marks, however, are frequently found on more accessible areas such as cheeks or arms.

Characters

Bite marks may indicate the character of the assault. Those inflicted during sexual assault often have central "suck" marks associated with them. Those inflicted during aggressive physical assault do not exhibit "suck" marks but have more "tool" mark appearances.

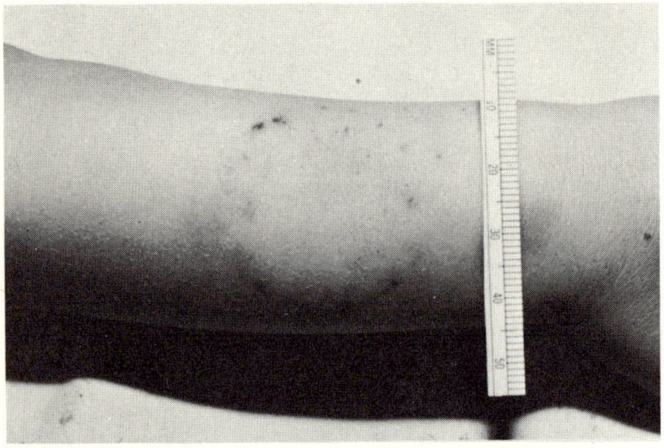

Figs. 6-5 to 6-8 Two brothers left in the care of a 19-year-old male babysitter were assaulted. One child lived, the other died. Figs. 6-5 and 6-6 show bite mark injuries on the arm of the murder victim. Fig. 6-7 shows a bite mark injury on the arm of the surviving brother. Fig. 6-8 is of a cigarette burn in the palm of the surviving child.

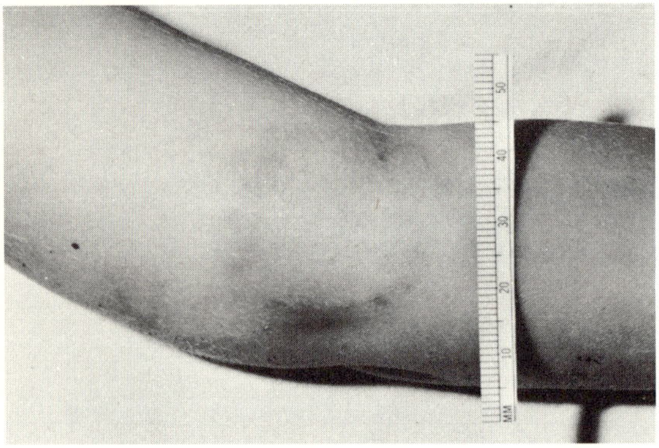

Figure 6-6

Considerations

Bite marks are mirror images of the dentitions that caused them. Documented cases have shown that human skin reflects the characteristics of teeth surprisingly well in certain cases.

Applying dental logic to bite mark interpretation can be fraught with danger. For instance, the absence of pattern marks for individual teeth sometimes occur, as does the absence of opposing arch marks. Positive evidence, the presence of marks, is much more valuable in drawing conclusions than negative evidence, the absence of marks.

Significance

Most often medical and/or dental evidence must speak for the abused child. The majority of these children are brought to hospital emergency rooms with histories of accidental traumas given by the parents or adult guardians. But bite mark injuries are seldom accidental and often indicate child abuse. Contrast with other

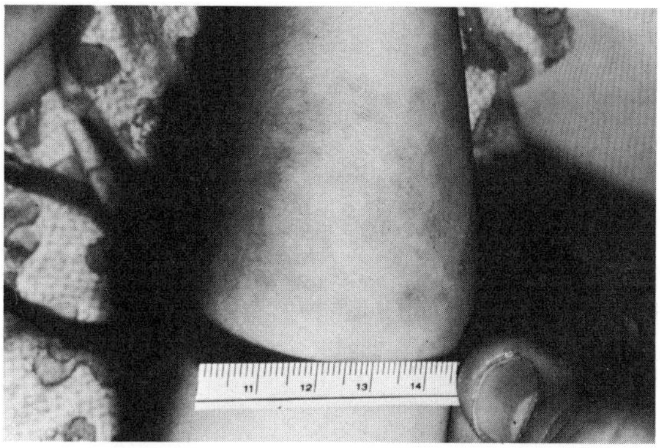

Figure 6-7

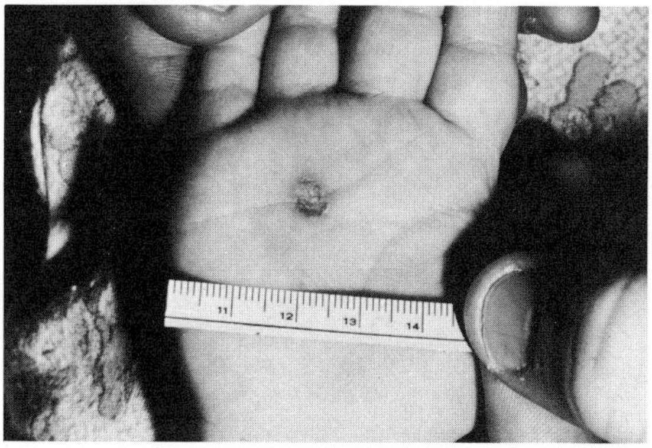

Figure 6-8

suspicious injuries, which can be difficult to prove nonaccidental with reasonable medical certainty.

Where bite mark evidence exists it is usually possible to exclude all but one person as the perpetrator. In most cases the person inflicting the bite marks has been the person responsible for physically abusing the child.

Documentation

The proper documentation of bite marks will be described in detail in Chapter 7. Suffice it to say here that documentation is similar on living and deceased children except that in deceased children tissue sections are taken for microscopic examination to date the injury. Since this obviously is not practical in the living child, special care must be taken to describe color changes in the injuries, and very accurate color photographs taken for age estimations by the forensic pathologist and odontologist.

Interpretation

The forensic odontologist attempts to answer certain questions in evaluating alleged bite mark injuries. The physician and dentist will find the following sequence useful for examination and diagnosis.

Is the Injury a Bite Mark?
- Ovoid or elliptical shape
- Size of arch
- Class characteristics of teeth
- Suck mark present/absent

Human or Animal Bite Mark?
- Presence of animal
- Arch form
- Arch size
- Perforation of canine areas
- Laceration and tissue tears
- Class characteristics of teeth
- ''Suck'' mark present/absent

Adult or Child Bite Mark?
- Arch size
- Class characteristic sizes of teeth

Upper or Lower Arch?
- Arch size
- Diffuse or distinct
- Class characteristics of incisor teeth

Which Teeth Represented?
- Class characteristics of teeth types

Individualization Possible?
- Unique and individual characteristics

Bite Marks and Other Trauma Contemporaneous?
- Color changes
- Microscopic considerations

Referral

When it is decided that an injury pattern is indeed a human bite mark the implications become quite serious, for there is great likelihood that the case will be referred to the criminal justice system. Correct identification of the possible perpetrator and time relationship to the assault or homicide become crucial.

Bite mark investigation and comparison is a special skill requiring training and experience. While lack of training and experience need not preclude successful comparison of a bite mark injury with the teeth of possible perpetrators, the record mitigates against this. Because of the potential tragic consequences of mistakes by novices, and the worldwide availability of competent forensic odontologists, the risk is not worth the reward.

The forensic odontologist will usually examine photographs of the bite mark for all the unique and individual dentition characteristics that are reflected on the skin. He/she also will examine models of the teeth of all persons who have access to the child. These models are obtained by either informed consent or court order. They will be made by a licensed dentist according to accepted dental standards with a "chain of custody" preserved.

Techniques of comparison may vary depending on which the examiner finds most comfortable, and his conclusions, if any, will be reported either verbally or in writing.

References

Beckstead, J. W.; Rawson, R. D.; and Giles, W. S.: Review of Bite Mark Evidence. J. Am. Dent. Assoc. 99:69, 1979.

Levine, L. J.: The Solution of a Battered Child Homicide by Dental Evidence, Report of Case. J. Am. Dent. Assoc. 87:1234, 1973.

Levine, L. J.: Bite Mark Evidence. Dent. Clin. North Am. 21:145, 1977.

Sims, B. G.; Grant, J. H.; Cameron, J. M.: Bite Marks in the Battered Baby Syndrome. Med. Sci. Law, 13:207, 1973.

Sopher, I. M.: Forensic Dent. Springfield, Ill.: C.C. Thomas, 1976.

Sopher, I. M.: The Dentist and the Battered Child Syndrome. Dent. Clin. North Am. 21:113, 1977.

Woolridge, E. D.: Legal Problems of the Forensic Odontologist. J. For. Sci. 18:40, 1973.

An Atlas of Physical Child Abuse

Roger G. Sanger

The following atlas is presented to supplement Chapters 3–6 and to aid the clinician in the diagnosis of physical child abuse, especially to the craniofacial complex, neck, and upper extremities.

The following are acknowledged for their contributions:

The C. Henry Kempe National Center for the Prevention and Treatment of Child Abuse and Neglect
The American Academy of Pediatrics (Barton D. Schmitt, M.D.)
Stephen M. Blain, D.D.S.
Paul S. Casamassimo, D.D.S.
Ronald Johnson, D.D.S.
Eugene L. Keller, M.D.
Paul E. Kittle, D.D.S.
Howard L. Needleman, D.M.D.
Charles Poland, III, D.D.S.
David S. Richardson, D.D.S.
Patricia C. Tarren, D.D.S.
Paul O. Walker, D.D.S.
Gary A. Wilson, D.D.S.

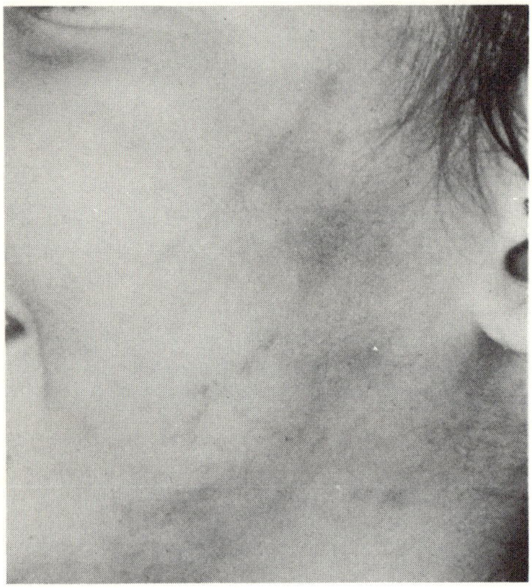

Fig. 1 Multiple bruises on the cheek representing pattern injury from adult hand slapped across the area.

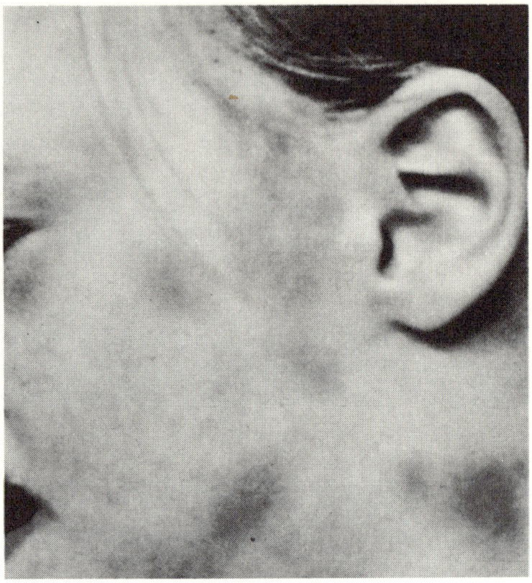

Fig. 2 Multiple bruises on the face and neck in different stages of resolution.

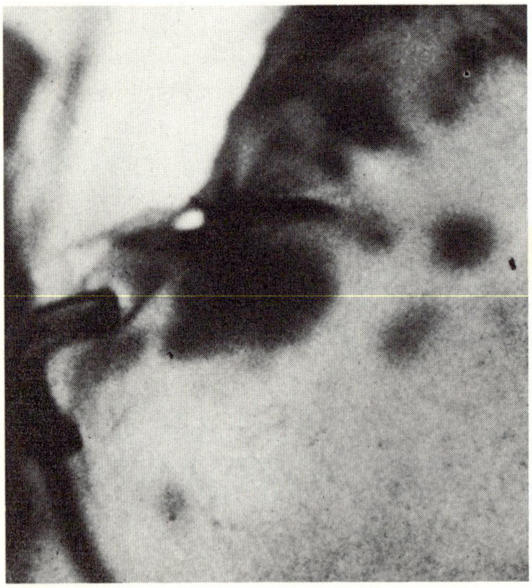

Fig. 3 Multiple bruises to the facial region in different stages of resolution. Child was hospitalized for subdural hematoma.

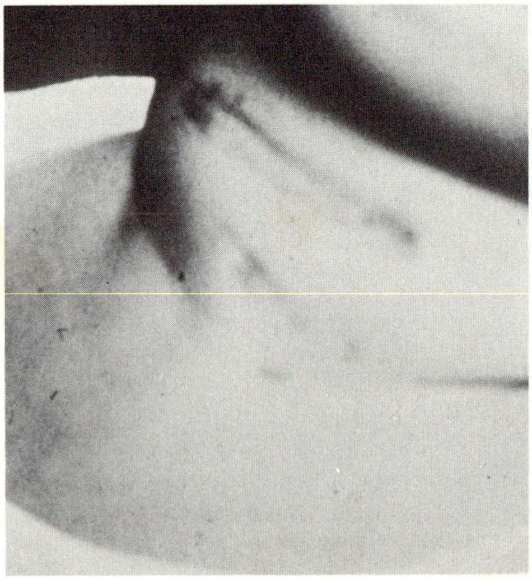

Fig. 4 Multiple bruises on the neck representing pattern injury from physical restraint (cord, rope, etc.) or attempted strangulation.

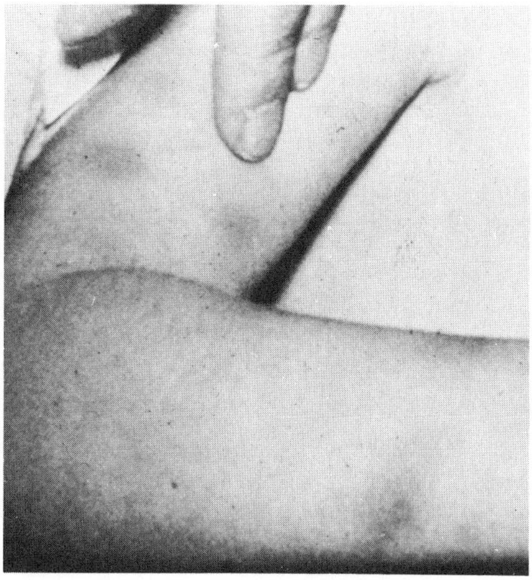

Fig. 5 Multiple bruises on the arm in different stages of resolution on a child with facial bruising.

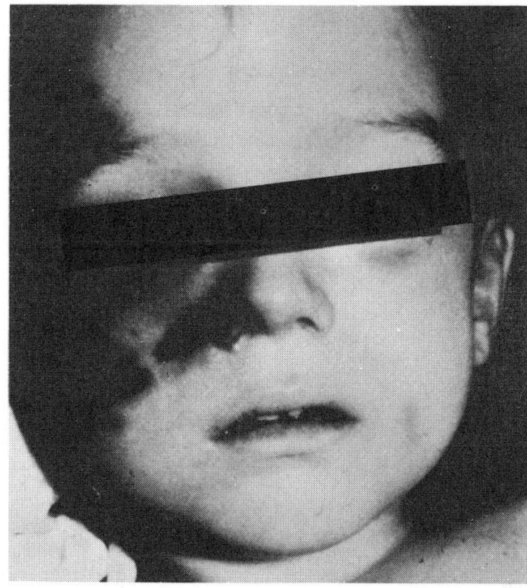

Fig. 6 Multiple lacerations and bruises on the face.

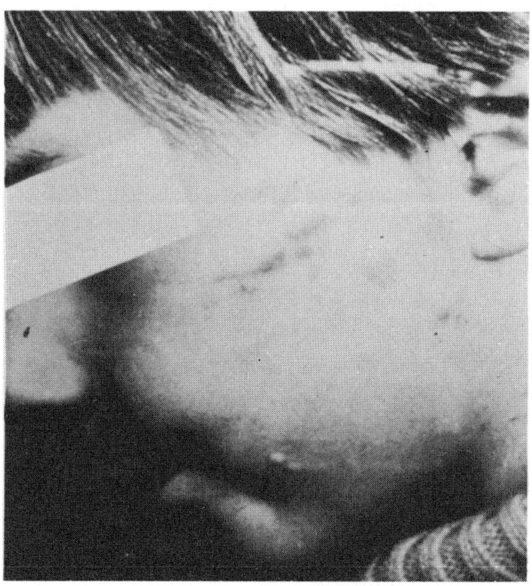

Fig. 7 Multiple lacerations on the cheek representing pattern injury from adult hand slapping.

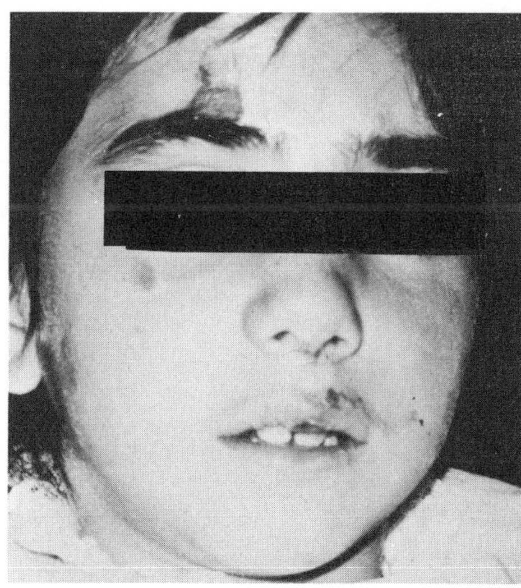

Fig. 8 Multiple lacerations on the face in different stages of resolution.

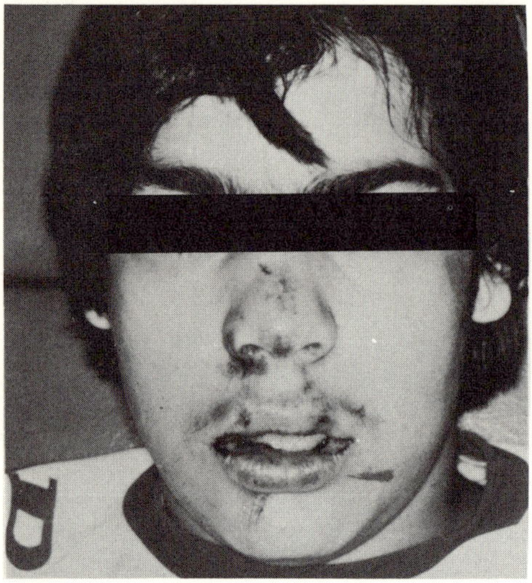

Fig. 9 Multiple lacerations on the face representing pattern injury from instrument.

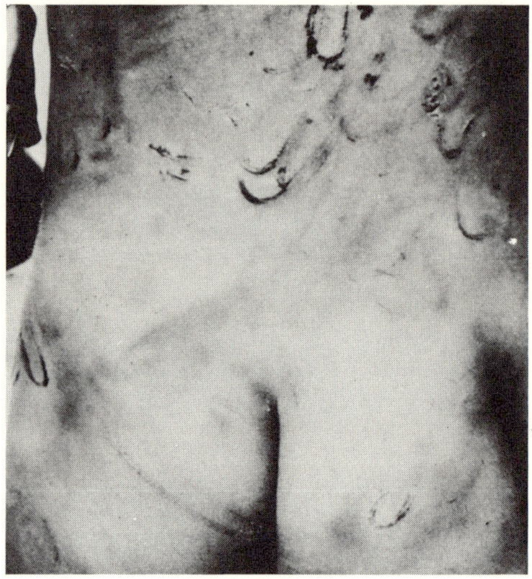

Fig. 10 Multiple lacerations, bruises, and bite marks on the back, buttocks, and legs in different stages of resolution and in areas not accessible to self-infliction. Pattern injury from looped instrument is represented.

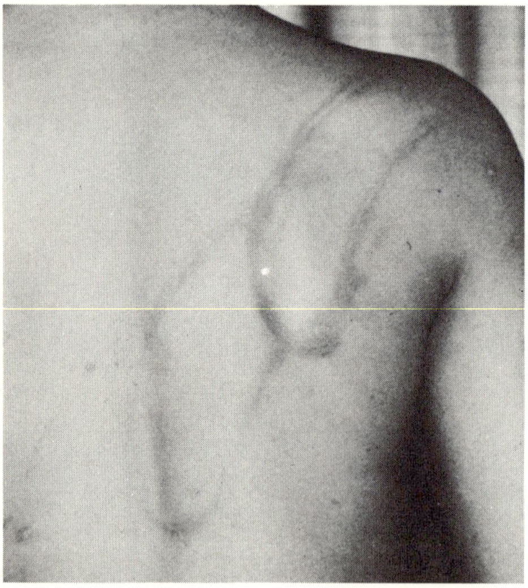

Fig. 11 Multiple bruises on the back representing pattern injury from loop instrument (cord, coat hanger, belt, etc.).

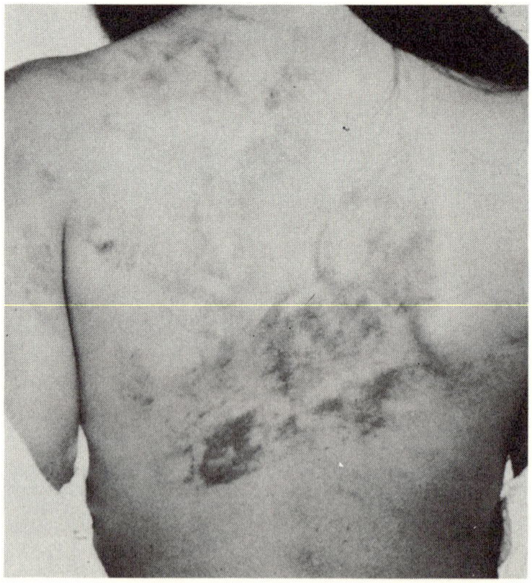

Fig. 12 Multiple bruises on the back in different stages of resolution representing pattern injury.

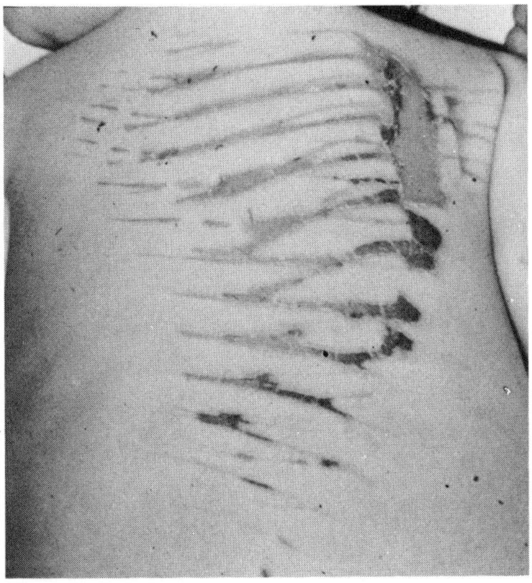

Fig. 13 Multiple lacerations and burns on the back representing pattern injury with hot instrument.

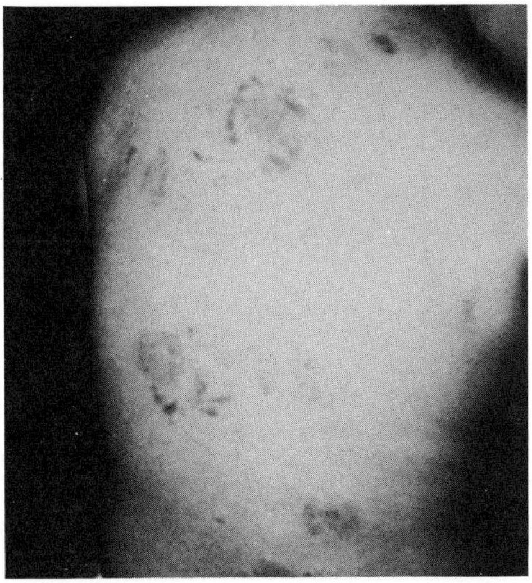

Fig. 14 Multiple bite marks (bruises and punctures) on the back.

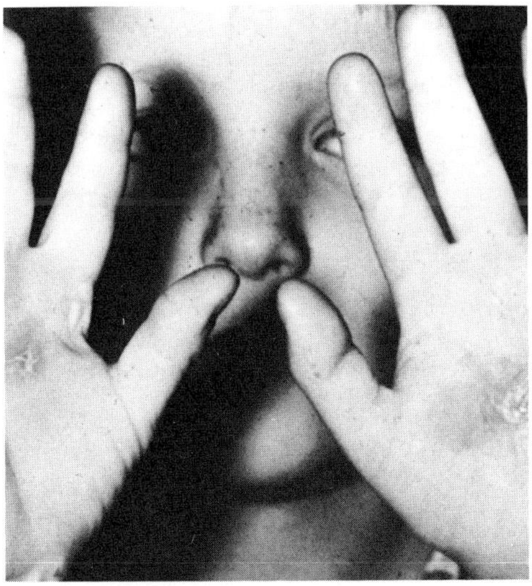

Fig. 15 Burns in the palm of hand representing pattern injury from hot, blunt instrument (cigar, cigarette, utensil, etc.).

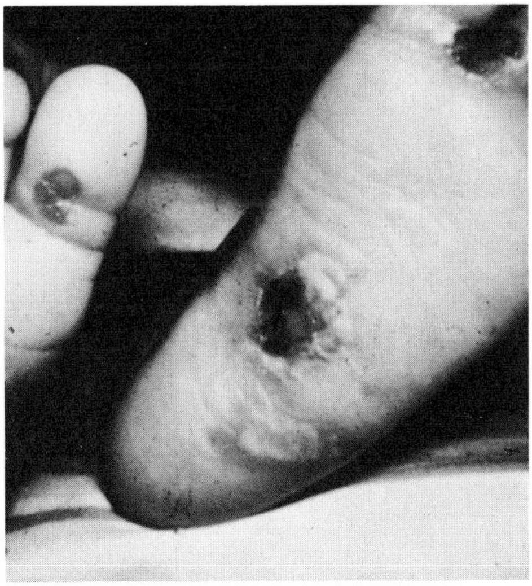

Fig. 16 Multiple burns on soles of feet in different stages of resolution and representing pattern injury from hot, blunt instrument (cigar, cigarette, utensil, etc.).

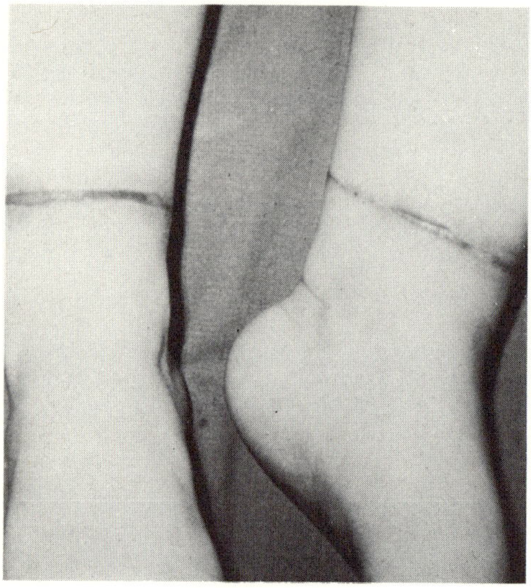

Fig. 17 Circumferential lacerations of the ankles representing pattern injury from physical restraints (cord, rope, etc.).

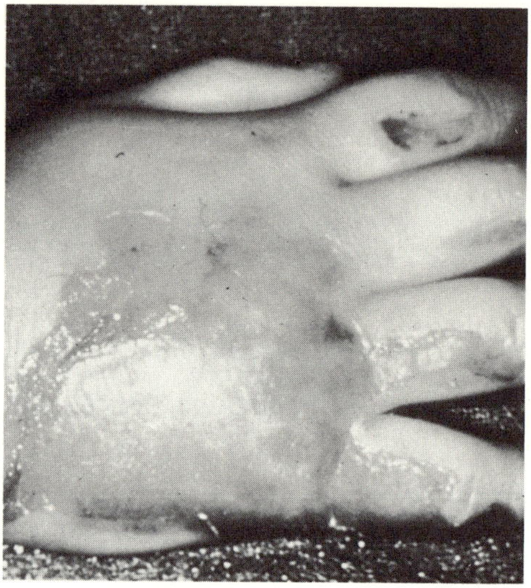

Fig. 18 Burns of the hand representing immersion in hot liquid.

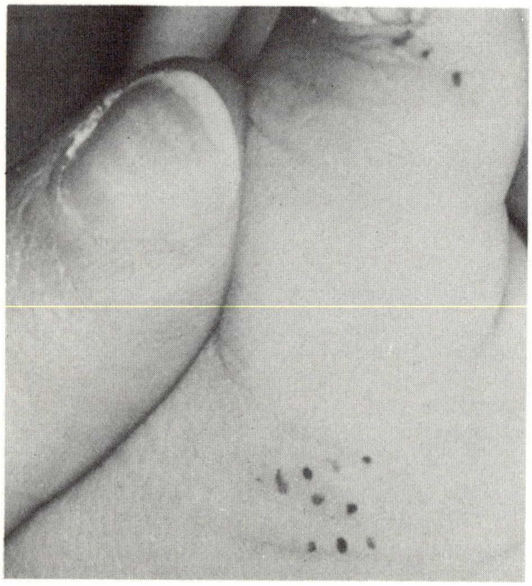

Fig. 19 Multiple puncture wounds on the hand representing pattern injury from sharp instrument.

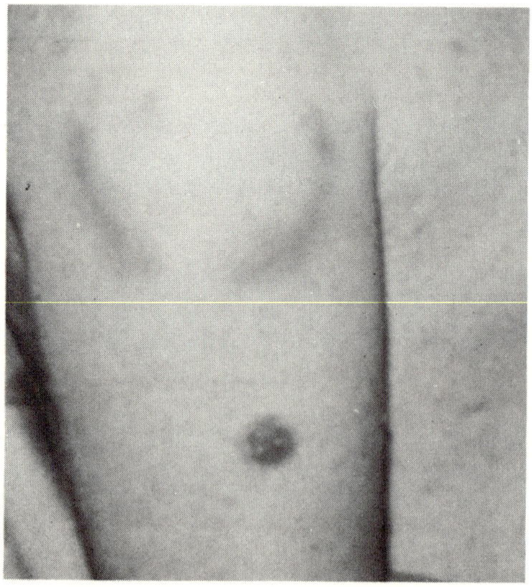

Fig. 20 Bruises and bite mark (bruises) on the arm.

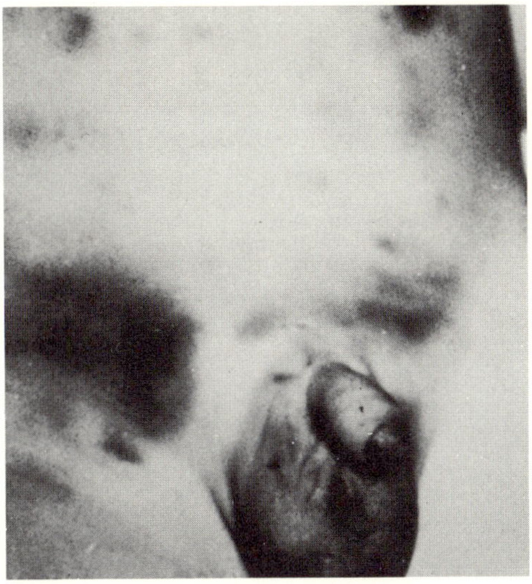

Fig. 21 Multiple bruises on the abdomen and genitalia.

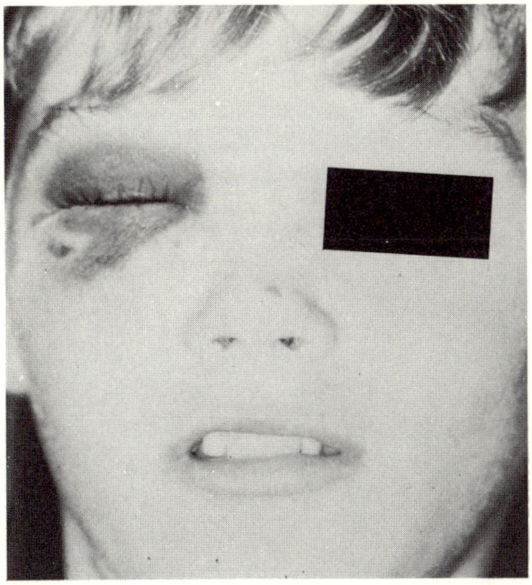

Fig. 22 Bruising and swelling to the orbital area representing trauma with blunt force.

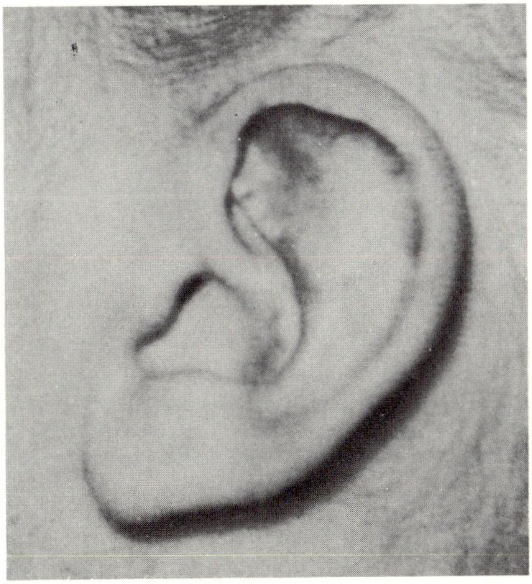

Fig. 23 Bruising and swelling to the ear.

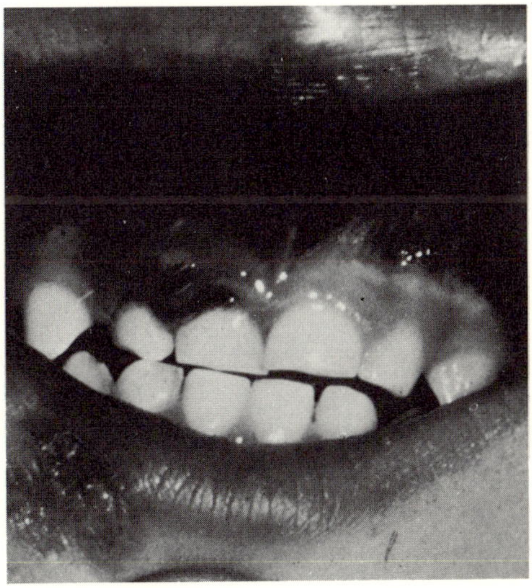

Fig. 24 Bruising and laceration to the lips and upper vestibule.

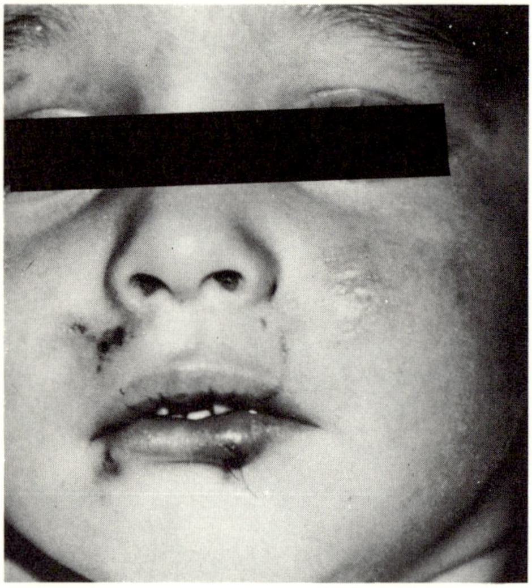

Figs. 26 and 27 Multiple bruises and lacerations to the face with laceration to maxillary vestibules and injury to the primary dentition.

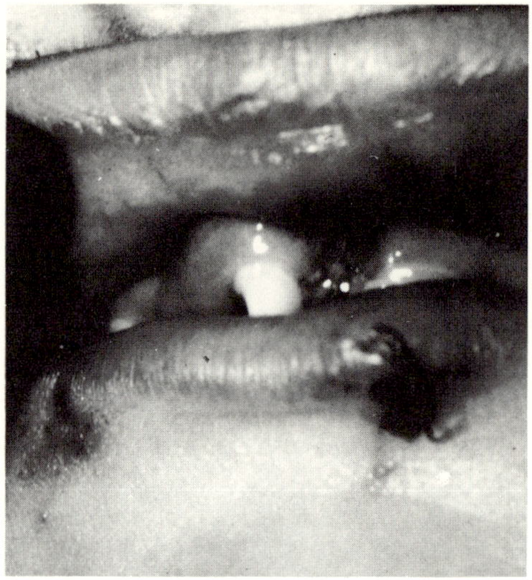

Figure 27

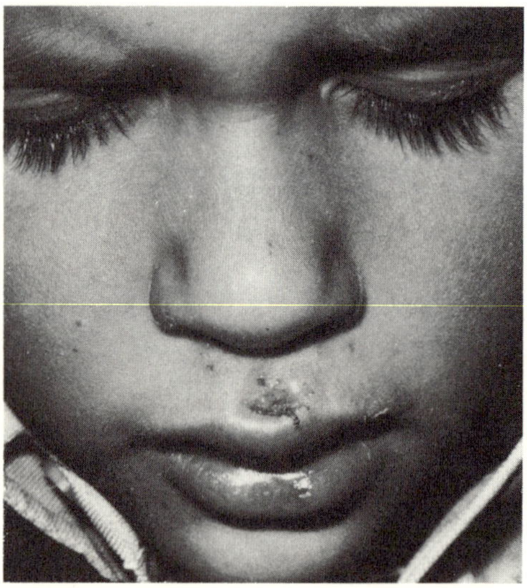

Figs. 28 and 29 Lacerations to the upper lip and upper vestibule.

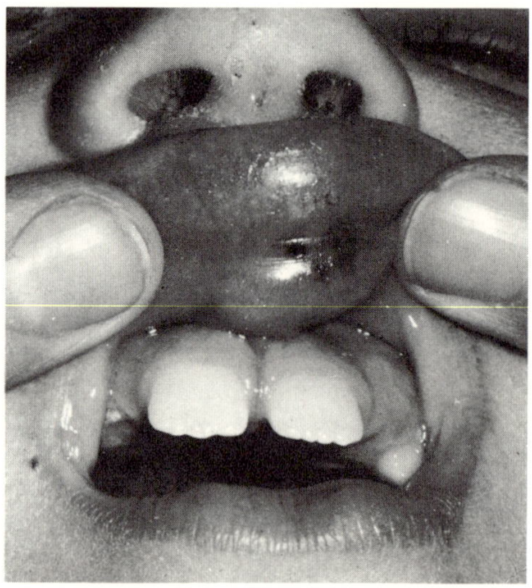

Figure 29

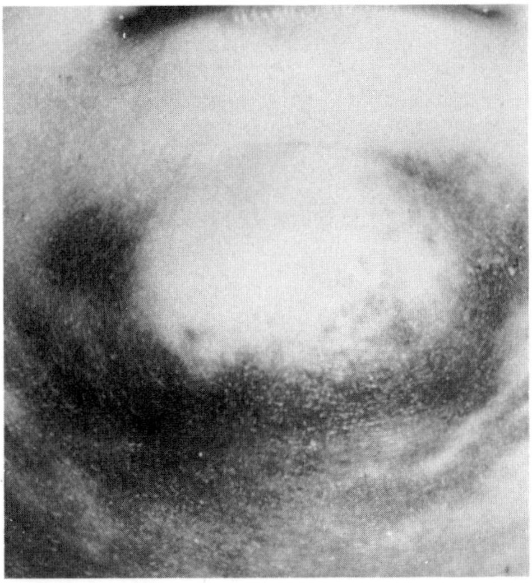

Fig. 30 Circumferential bruising to the chin representing pattern injury of circular object (cup, large ring, etc.).

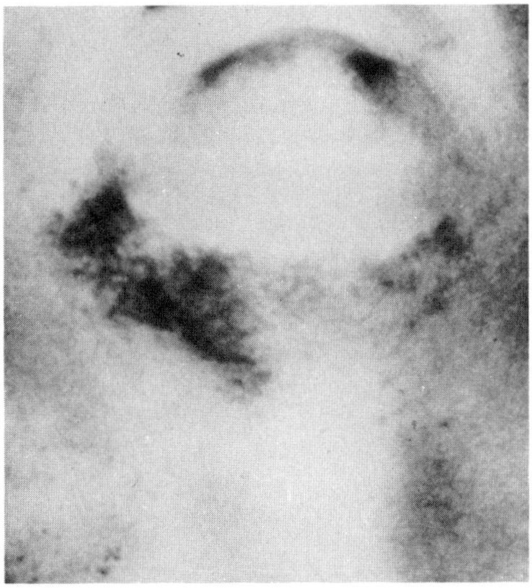

Fig. 31 Semicircular bruising to the chin representing pattern injury from semicircular object.

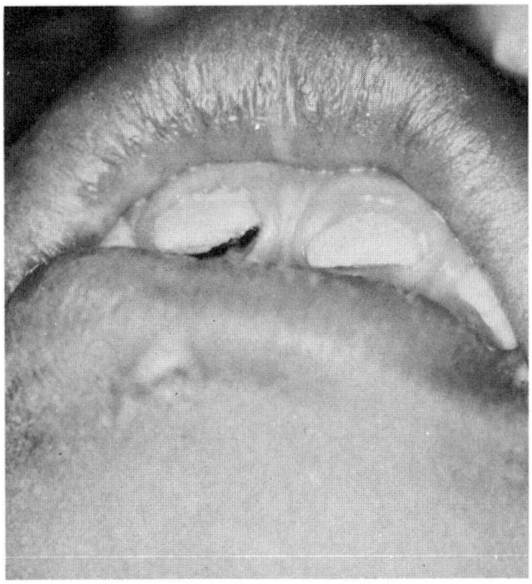

Figs. 32 and 33 Laceration to the lower lip and vestibule with presence of injury to maxillary incisor. Patient had history of convulsive disorder and gingival hyperplasia.

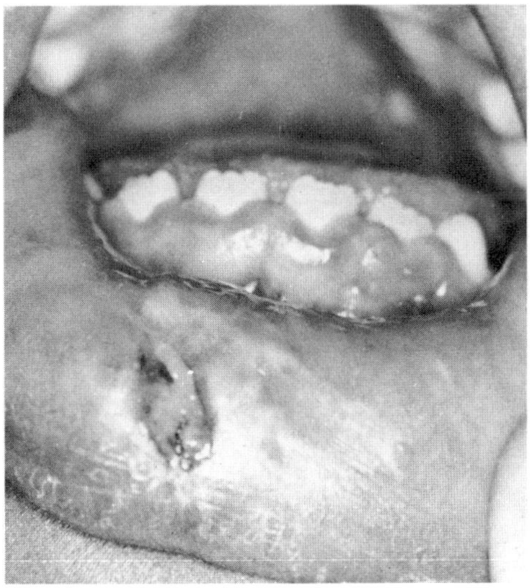

Figure 33

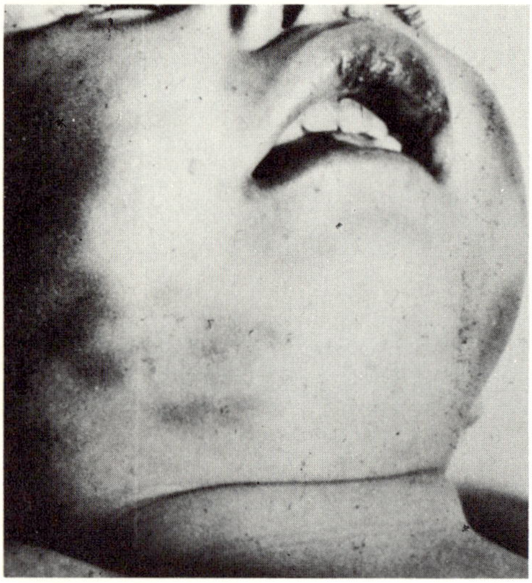

Fig. 34 Bruising and swelling to upper lip and vestibule combined with bruises of the neck representing pattern injury from adult hand pressure, possibly indicating forced feeding with blunt instrument (spoon, etc.).

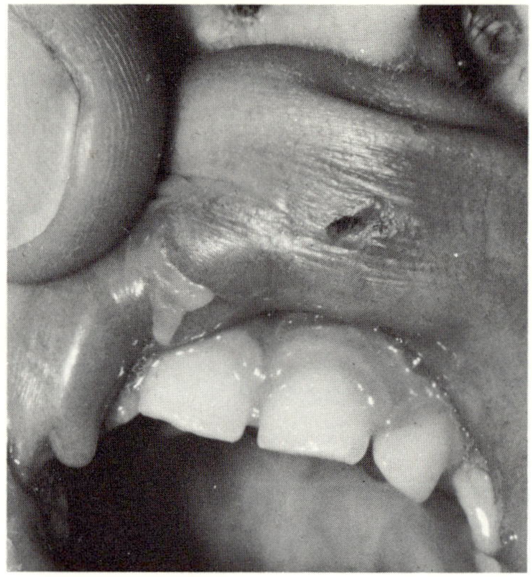

Fig. 35 Multiple lacerations (puncture wounds) to vestibules representing pattern injury from sharp, pronged instrument (fork, etc.).

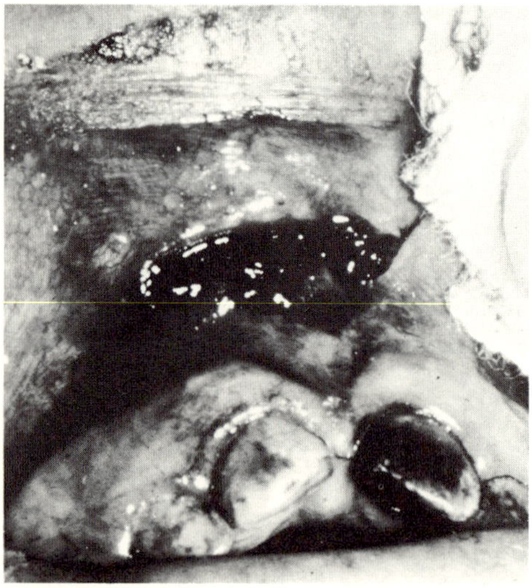

Fig. 36 Laceration to the maxillary frenum with previous injury to the dentition.

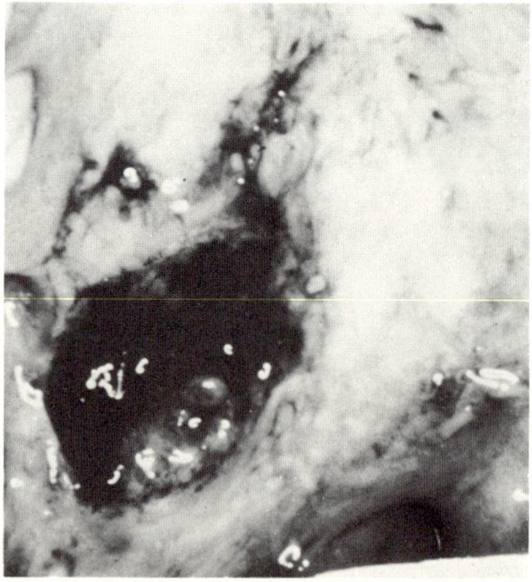

Fig. 37 Multiple laceration (puncture wounds) on the palate representing pattern injury from sharp instrument (knife, etc.).

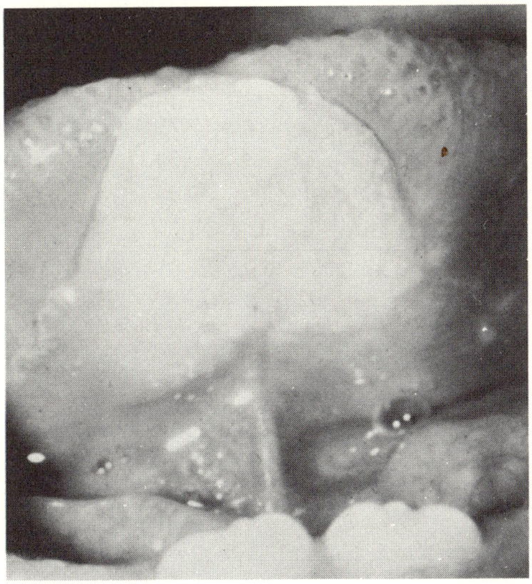

Fig. 38 Large burn on under surface of tongue representing pattern injury from hot, blunt instrument (spoon, etc.).

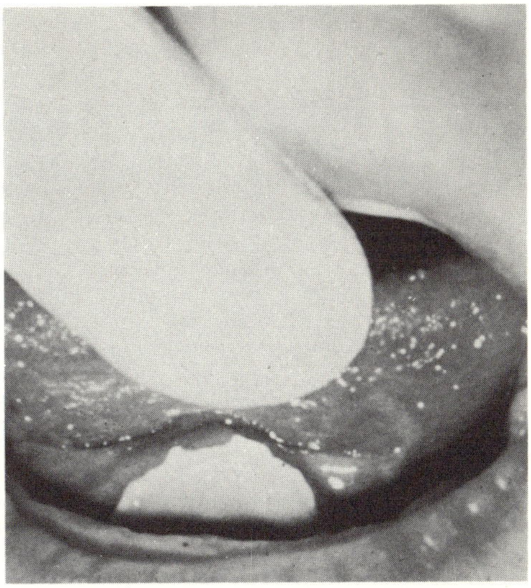

Fig. 39 Large burn on floor of mouth combined with burns to nose.

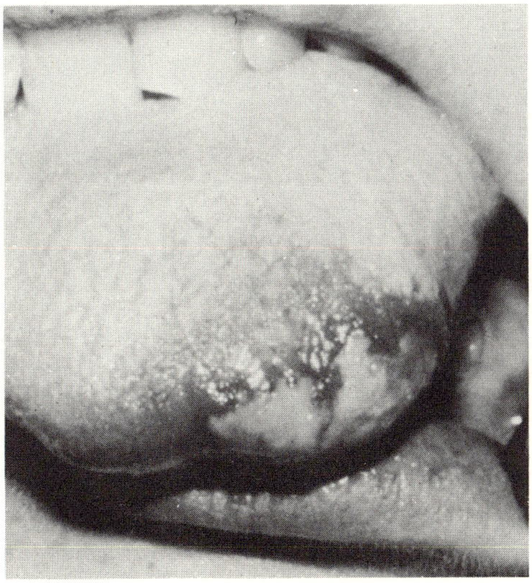

Fig. 40 Burn and swelling to tip of tongue.

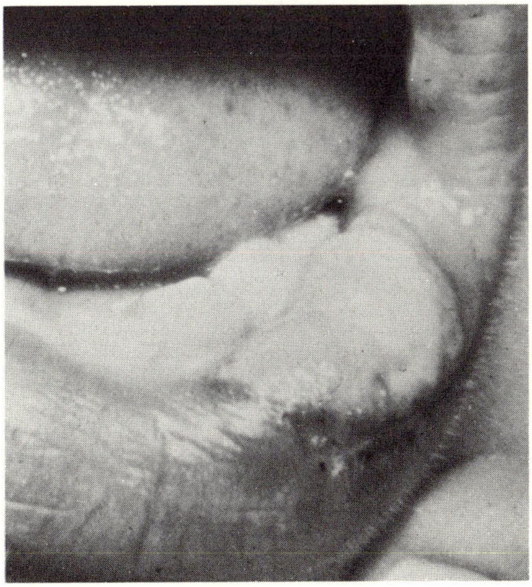

Fig. 41 Burn to lower lip.

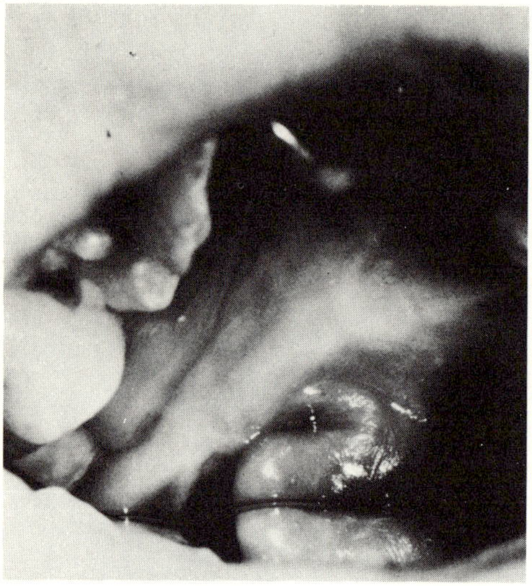

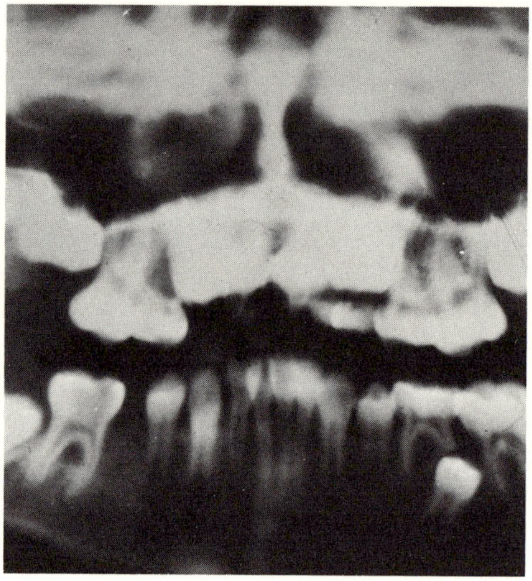

Figs. 42 and 43 Constricture of oral musculature and severe malocclusion resulting from repeated placement of caustic chemical in mouth.

Figure 43

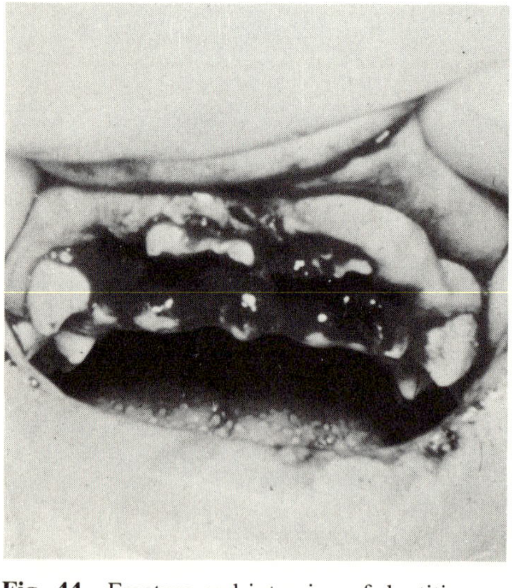

Fig. 44 Fracture and intrusion of dentition.

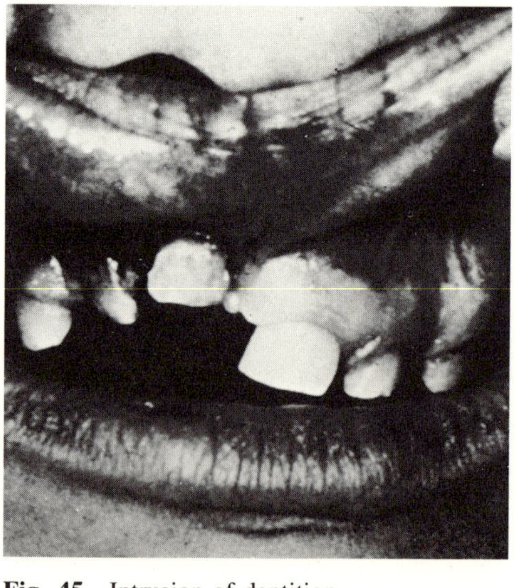

Fig. 45 Intrusion of dentition.

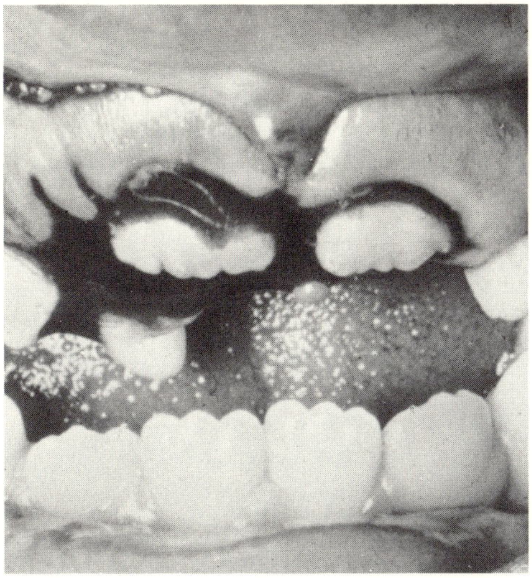

Fig. 46 Partial avulsion of dentition.

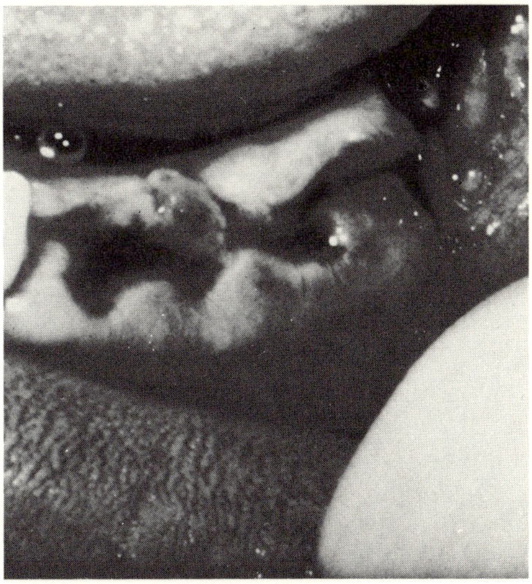

Figs. 47 to 49 Avulsion of numerous teeth in the lower jaw representing blunt force.

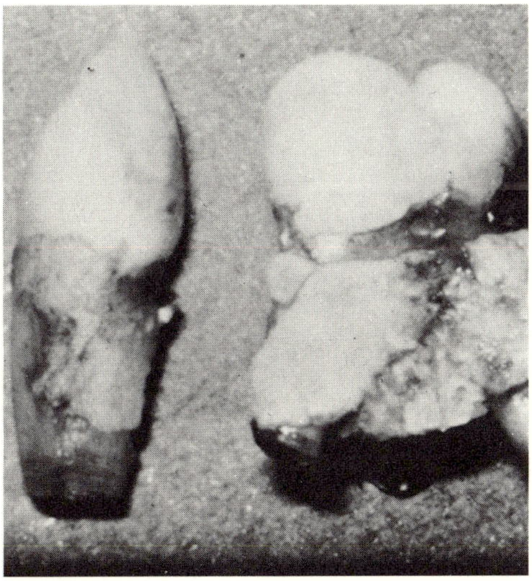

Figure 48

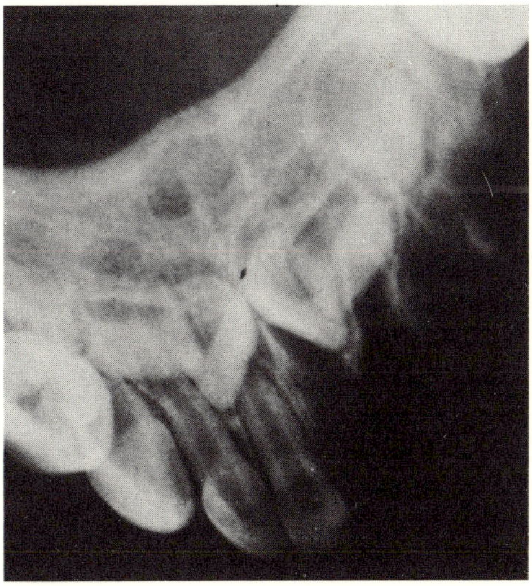

Figure 49

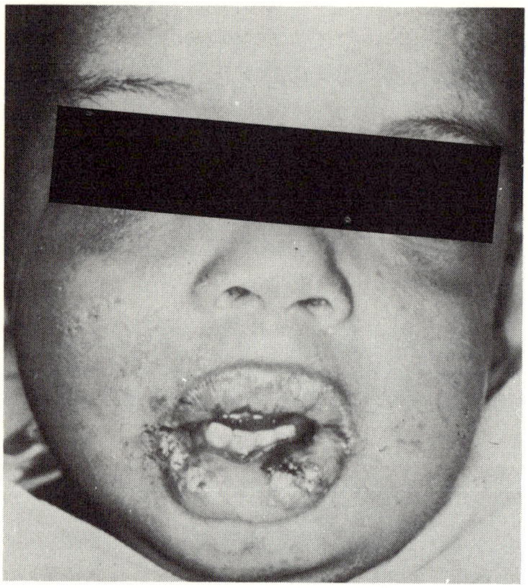

Figs. 50 to 53 Multiple lacerations and swelling of face, fracture of symphysis of the lower jaw, nasal injury, and bruising to the upper vestibule.

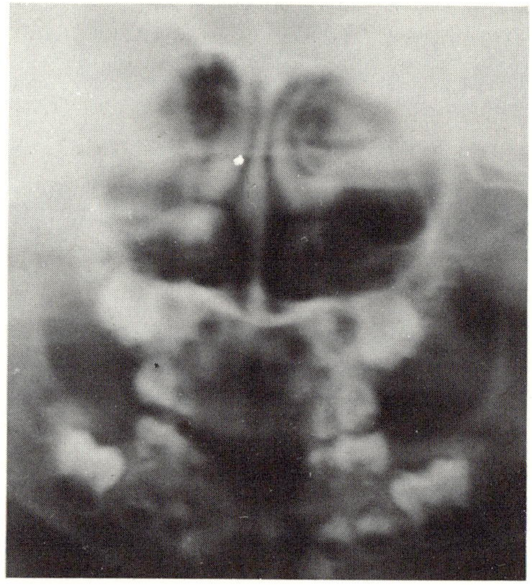

Figure 51

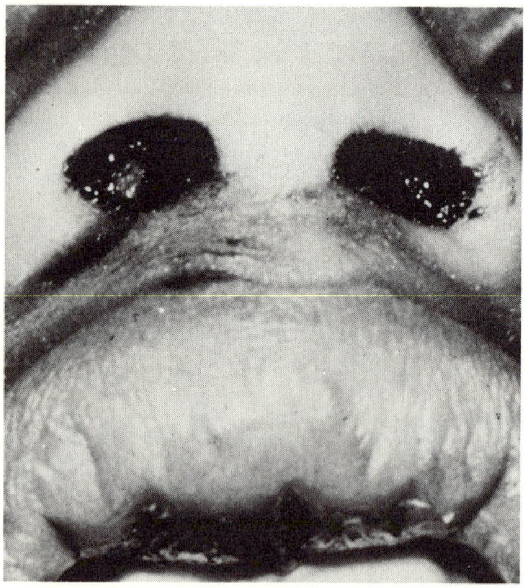

Figure 52

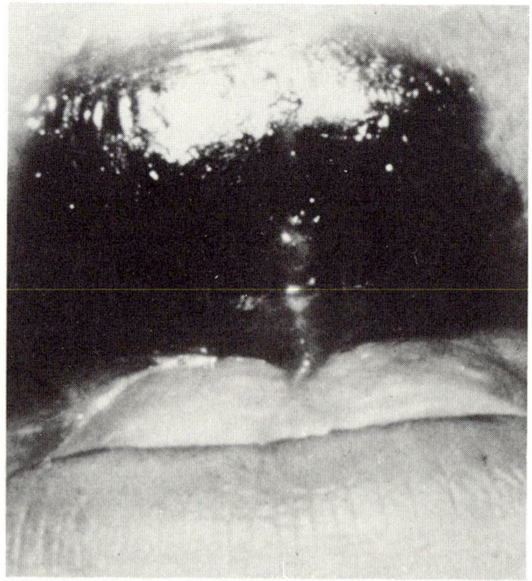

Figure 53

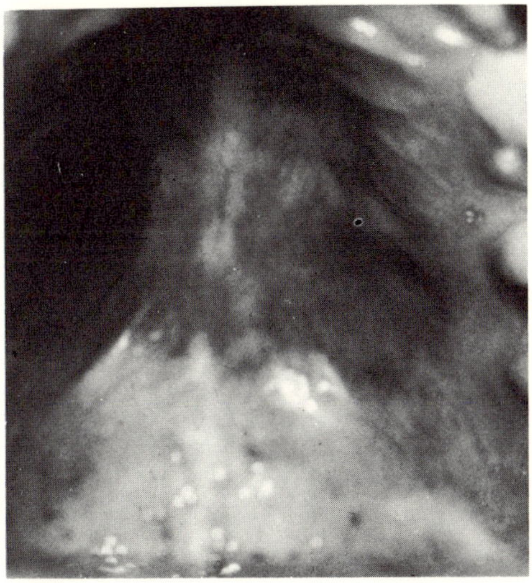

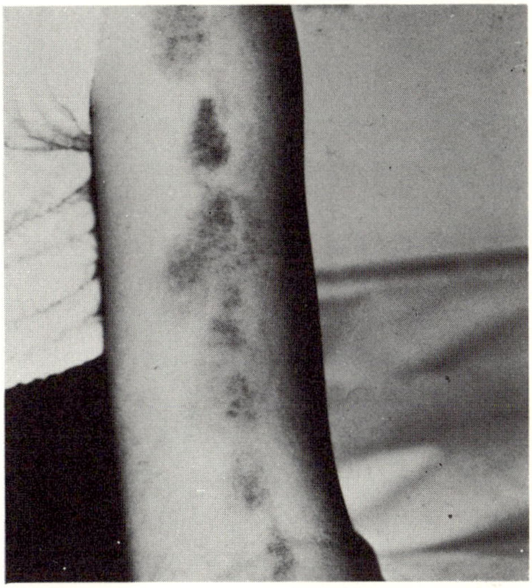

Figs. 54 and 55 Multiple petechiae of the palate combined with multiple bite and sucking marks on the area representing self-inflicted injury.

Figure 55

Chapter 7

Documentation and Collection of Physical Evidence

Roger G. Sanger

Introduction

One of the most important yet often overlooked responsibilities of the dental professional who suspects child abuse or neglect is the systematic documentation and collection of physical evidence. This is essential for proper identification and diagnosis.

No matter how thoroughly an examination has been performed, it is of little value unless the findings are recorded permanently and accurately for proper evaluation and detailed comparison at a later date when they might be needed as evidence in court (DeVore, 1977).

Dental Evidence

Dental evidence carries no special significance in the court because it is scientific. It may be challenged, disbelieved, or rejected the same as nonscientific evidence. Scientific evidence can offer certainty only within the limits of human experience. When scientific evidence is beyond the scope of judicial knowledge it must be personally attested to by one or more experts (Brownlie, 1976). Because dental evidence in suspected cases of child abuse is rarely within the scope of judicial knowledge and is often limited by human experience, its documentation, collection, evaluation, and explanation by experts must be of the highest standard. In many cases, documentation and collection of dental evidence may be accomplished by one expert but evaluated and explained by other experts. This gives prime importance to the proper documentation and collection of physical evidence by the first dental professional.

Documentation and Collection

Documentation and collection of physical evidence requires a systematic approach and the use of a permanent, accurate, and reproducible record. Recording techniques include but are not limited to: written observation, photographs, radiographs, and cast models. Documentation and collection of physical evidence requires, by definition, a thorough examination process. Because the dental professional may encounter injuries of physical abuse, lesions of sexual abuse, and bite marks in cases of suspected child abuse, the following will serve as guidelines for the documentation and collection of physical evidence in each of these clinical situations. It is important to remember that these are only guidelines and that individual circumstances may dictate deviation. However, since one or more experts may be attesting to dental evidence documented and collected by another expert, standardization should be observed where possible. The chain of evidence collection and custody must be in agreement with accepted standards and state statutes.

The Examination Process

When the dental professional is confronted with a case of suspected child abuse, it is essential that a thorough examination appropriate for the dental office be performed and all physical evidence documented and collected before proceeding with treatment and interview. Although dental professionals should screen all their child patients for signs of abuse, more definitive examinations should be performed when suspicion exists (Kittle et al., 1981).

A definitive examination on child patients suspected of being abused should include but not be limited to the following areas, using a systems approach:

- Head and neck region including scalp, eyes, ears, nose, and mouth
- Body surfaces both exposed and covered, within the limits of accepted dental practice
- Body organs within the limits of accepted dental practice

Another dental office staff member should be present during all definitive child abuse examination procedures. This person should be told of the suspicion before examination, and may serve as legal witness as well as recorder of the dental professional's observations (Kittle et al., 1981).

Injuries From Physical Abuse

Injuries of physical abuse in the oral facial region should be documented as follows:

1. Written Observations

With a dental office staff member present as either recorder or nonrecording observer, a detailed description of the injury(s) should be recorded in ink in the patient's dental record. Legible, intelligible transcription and appropriate diagrams and drawings are encouraged. The injury or injuries should be described by:

- Number
- Type (bruise, laceration, puncture, etc.)
- Size (diameter, length, depth, etc.)
- Location (soft tissue, bony involvement, etc.)

- Resolution (date of approximate occurrence)
- Possible causes (e.g., pattern injury from utensil)
- Opinions

Injuries observed on other body surfaces/organs within accepted dental practice should be similarly recorded, and all transcriptions dated and signed by examiner and recorder.

2. Photographs

When available, 35-mm color photographs of the injury(s) are invaluable. They should be taken with metric rulers, identification labels, and color scales focused at or near the injury. The identification tag should note patient name, date, film type, and technician name. Numerous photographs should be taken from different angles and bracketed with different film exposures, which also should be recorded. Photographs of injury(s) observed on other body surfaces/organs within dental practice are encouraged.

3. Radiographs

Although the injury(s) might not involve hard tissue (bones and teeth), it is often appropriate to obtain a full mouth radiographic and, if possible, panoramic survey to determine the presence of recent or old hard tissue injury. Radiographs should not be altered (cut), and should be labelled with patient name, date, exposure, machine and film type, and technician name. Mounting of radiographs is encouraged.

4. Cast Models

If appropriate and necessary for preservation, an impression of the injury(s) can be taken using accepted dental materials and procedures. The impression should be processed as soon as possible and labelled with patient name, date, impression material used, cast material used, and technician name. Cast models are appropriate for evaluations of pattern injuries involving tissue destruction.

Lesions From Sexual Abuse

Oral facial lesions characteristic of sexually transmitted diseases should be documented as follows:

1. Written Observations

With a dental office staff member present as either recorder or nonrecording observer, detailed descriptions of the lesions should be recorded in ink in the patient's dental record. Legible, intelligible transcription and appropriate diagrams and drawings are encouraged. The lesions should be described by:

- Number
- Type (ulceration, petechiae, etc.)
- Size (diameter, length, depth, etc.)
- Location (soft tissue, bony involvement, etc.)
- Resolution (date of approximate occurrence)

- Possible causes (disease, trauma, etc.)
- Opinions

Lesions observed on other body surfaces/organs within accepted dental practice should be recorded in similar manner and all transcription dated and signed by examiner and recorder.

2. Photographs

Thirty-five-millimeter color photographs of the lesions are invaluable and highly encouraged. Metric rulers, identification labels, and color scales should be focused at or near the lesions. The same procedures as outlined for photographing physical abuse injuries should be followed when photographing lesions from suspected sexual abuse.

3. Radiographs and Cast Models

For the same reasons as for physical abuse injuries, radiographs and cast models of lesions from suspected sexual abuse are often appropriate. They should be accomplished using the same procedures as those outlined for physical abuse injuries.

Bite Marks

Marks indicative of a bite(s) on body parts where examination is within accepted dental practice (face, arms, legs, etc.) should be documented. Since it is likely that a forensic odontologist will be evaluating this evidence, as bite marks are often used by the courts for inclusion or exclusion of child abusers, abundant protocol for documenting bite marks is available. It can be generalized as follows (Luntz and Luntz, 1973; Sopher, 1976; Harvey, 1976; Levine, 1977; Sognnaes, 1977; Beckstead et al., 1979): If the dental professional is unsure whether markings on the body surface represent bites and/or whether they are caused by human, animal, or other means, it is appropriate to document what is observed in the dental office. Forensic odontologists can make these discriminations later from well-documented and well-collected evidence.

1. Written Observations

With a dental staff member present as either recorder or nonrecording observer, detailed descriptions of the markings should be recorded in ink in the patient's dental record. Legible, intelligible transcription and appropriate diagrams and drawings are encouraged. Each marking should be described by:

- Number
- Type (bruise, laceration, puncture, sucking marks, etc.)
- Size (diameter or dimension of ovoid markings)
- Location
- Resolution (date of approximate occurrence)
- Possible causes (adult, child, animal, other)
- Opinions

All transcription should be dated and signed by examiner and recorder.

2. Photographs
Thirty-five-millimeter color and black and white contrast photographs are invaluable. They should be taken with metric rulers, identification labels, and color scales focused at or near the markings. The identification tag should include patient name, date, film type, and technician name. Several photographs should be taken from different angles and bracketed with different film exposures, which also should be recorded. Photographs of the complete body surfaces where markings occurred, and of the markings themselves without rulers, identification labels, and color scales also are suggested.

3. Radiographs
Radiographic survey is not useful for bite mark analysis unless the bite marks are concomitant with injuries of physical abuse and/or lesions of sexual abuse.

4. Saliva Sampling
If proper equipment is available and skill in the procedure established, the dental professional should swab the involved skin to check for secretory antigens conveyed by the saliva of the biter. Approximately 80 percent secrete are the basic A, B, and O blood group protein antigenic complexes concentrated in whole saliva.

Although actual testing is performed in a forensic laboratory, a dental professional can swab with a sterile cotton swab moistened with isotonic saline solution. The examiner removes the sterile swab from the sealed container (vial), moistens it, swabs the skin, and replaces it into the container. A control sample should be taken from another body surface of the patient.

A saliva sample from the patient should be stored in a sealable container (vial). Dried saliva on the bite does not necessarily eliminate the detection process. Samples should be tested in the forensic laboratory as soon as possible after collection. Only uncontaminated portions of the markings should be swabbed. Although useful, the technique is not infallible.

5. Cast Models
If sufficient tissue destruction exists from bite marks, impressions of the markings can be taken using accepted dental materials and procedures. Rubber-base or silicone impression materials are preferred. To support the impression material before it is removed from the body surface, it is necessary to apply a backing of dental stone, plaster, or other suitable material. More than one impression can be taken. They should be processed with accepted dental materials as soon as possible and labelled with patient name, date, impression material used, cast material used, and technician name.

Bite mark investigation is difficult and requires considerable training and experience in forensic odontology. The dental professional without this should not proceed without consulting a forensic odontologist.

Consent

In cases of suspected child abuse, parent/guardian informed consent is not mandatory for the previously described procedures. General consent to perform diagnostic procedures should be obtained just as it is for all children about to undergo dental examinations. No special consent is needed for any of these procedures for documenting cases of suspected child abuse, because they are all diagnostic in nature.

Custody of Evidence

Documented physical evidence should not be altered or left in an open-access location where alteration can occur. Evidence should be kept under locked conditions until properly processed by law enforcement, district attorney, or court agencies. The custody, processing, and transportation of evidence (chain of evidence) must be correct and upheld to the highest judicial standards in order to be presentable and acceptable to the courts. State statutes will dictate these procedures.

Summary

The dental professional may need to document and collect physical evidence from patients who are suspected victims of child abuse. Injuries of physical abuse, lesions of sexual abuse, and bite marks dictate certain standards of documentation and collection for the evidence to be evaluated by experts and presented to courts.

Acknowledgment

The author wishes to thank Homer R. Campbell, Jr., for his assistance in the preparation of this chapter.

References

Beckstead, J. W.; Rawson, R. D.; and Giles, W. S.: Review of Bite Mark Evidence. J. Am. Dent. Assoc. 99:69, 1979.

Brownlie, A. R.: Legal Aspects of Forensic Odontology. In Harvey, W. Dental Identification and Forensic Odontology. London: Henry Kimpton, 1976, p. 168.

DeVore, D. T.: Radiology and Photography in Forensic Dentistry. Dent. Clin. North Am. 21:69, 1977.

Harvey, W.: Dental Identification and Forensic Odontology. London: Henry Kimpton, 1976, pp. 88, 124.

Kittle, P. E.; Richardson, D. S.; and Parker, J. W.: Two Child Abuse/Child Neglect Examinations for the Dentist. J. Dent. Child. 48:175, 1981.

Levine, L. J.: Bite Mark Evidence. Dent. Clin. North Am. 21:145, 1977.

Luntz, L. L. and Luntz, P.: Handbook for Dental Identification. Philadelphia: Lippincott, 1973, p. 148.

Sognnaes, R. F.: The Case for Better Bite and Bite Mark Preservations. Int. J. For. Dent. 4:17, 1977.

Sopher, I. M.: Forensic Dentistry. Springfield: C.C. Thomas, 1976, p. 125.

Chapter 8

Treatment of Oral Facial Injuries and Lesions in Child Abuse

Howard L. Needleman

Introduction

The treatment of orofacial injuries and lesions sustained in child abuse can only superficially be covered in this chapter. For a more comprehensive discussion of this topic, the reader should refer to texts on pediatric dentistry, oral surgery, and oral pathology, some of which are contained in the reference list.

Treatment Goals

A basic goal is to treat these injuries as definitively as possible during the initial visit. Once suspicion of child abuse is revealed to the parents and/or the appropriate referral agency, the quality of follow-up care might not be ideal.

If the initial examination reveals trauma limited to the oral cavity and treatment is within the scope of the attending dentist, definitive treatment should commence. When treatment is completed, the dentist should discuss with the accompanying adult treatment rendered, prognosis, necessary follow-up care, and the symptoms of more serious head injury that they should look for (see chapter appendix). Once this has been accomplished, the issue of suspected child abuse should be discussed.

If, however, the examination reveals trauma beyond the attending dentist's ability to treat, he or she can perform limited initial emergency treatment before making an appropriate referral. In cases of severe trauma to the alveoli, jaws, or intraoral soft tissues, an oral surgeon is best qualified to provide treatment. Facial lacerations requiring extensive suturing might best be treated by a plastic surgeon. Unfamiliar oral lesions can be referred to an oral pathologist, oral surgeon, or pedodontist. Trauma involving the body, neurological system or extremities must always be treated by a physician, in either a private or an institutional setting. Initial treatment must be completed and these referrals made before discussing the issue of child abuse with the parents or guardians, since referral recommendations and follow-ups can be jeopardized if parents or guardians feel threatened.

Factors in Treatment Consideration

In treating children with orofacial injuries it is necessary to consider the following:

1. Child's Age and Ability to Cooperate
The dentist must first assess whether the patient is mature enough to cooperate with projected treatment modalities. Ideal treatment may have to be compromised or modified with an unmanageable child. Introduction of sedative premedication alone or in conjunction with nitrous oxide/oxygen analgesia and the use of physical restraints, such as a papoose board,[1] may be essential for management of the very young or very apprehensive patient. The parents or guardians should not be present in the room during treatment, as their presence may hinder communication with the distraught child.

2. Parental Attitudes
The attitudes of parents or caretakers toward dental care are sometimes a factor in treatment decisions. In cases where child abuse is suspected, parental input might not be sought. Instead, treatment approaches with the best prognoses should be selected. If risky or complex procedures are elected over more conservative or simple alternatives, chance of failure will increase due to possible lack of parental follow-up.

3. Dentition and General Health Conditions
Treatment considerations should also include: (a) space maintenance of primary units, (b) root development of involved teeth, (c) coronal development of the succedaneous teeth, (d) dental occlusion, and (e) medical status of the patient. Each of these variables can affect the treatment modalities selected (Craig and Hargreaves, 1981).

Child's Immunization Record
The patient's immunization status for tetanus must be ascertained. Primary immunization is achieved through the normal series of three DPT injections during childhood. An additional booster is recommended preferably at the time of entrance into school. Booster doses must be considered in wound management. A booster is required if the wound is particularly tetanus-prone (i.e., yielding anaerobic conditions or exposed to tetanus spores such as necrotizing machine injuries, puncture wounds, wounds heavily contaminated with extreta) and more than five years have passed since the last dose. Other wounds are considered low risk and a booster is necessary only if it is more than 10 years since the last dose (AAP, 1977). Table 8-1 recommends booster doses according to patient age and immunization status, and wound risk level.

[1]Olympic Papoose Board, Olympic Surgical Co., Seattle, Wash.

Table 8-1 Recommended use of tetanus toxoid and human tetanus-immune globulin (TIG) in wound management, determined by immunization status

Wound type	Booster dose
Unimmunized, uncertain, or incomplete (one or two doses of toxoid)	
Low-risk	One dose of Td* or DT† followed by completion of immunization; booster every 10 years thereafter.
Tetanus-prone and neglected for > 24 hours	One dose of Td* or DT† plus 250–500 units TIG followed by completion of immunization. Note: Use separate syringe and sites for TIG and toxoid.
Full primary immunization with booster dose within 10 years of wound	
Low-risk	No toxoid necessary.
Tetanus-prone	If > 5 years since last dose, one dose of Td*. If < 5 years, no toxoid necessary.
Neglected > 24 hours	One dose of Td* plus 250–500 units TIG.
Full primary immunization with no booster doses or last booster dose > 10 years	
Low-risk	One dose of Td*.
Tetanus-prone	One dose of Td*.
Neglected > 24 hours	One dose of Td* plus 250–500 units TIG.

*Td—adult. For patients > 6 years old.
†DT—pediatric. For patients < 6 years old.

Soft Tissue Injuries

Soft tissue injuries are the most common orofacial injury sustained in child abuse. Of these, contusions and ecchymoses, abrasions and lacerations, burns, fractures of the dentition, and human bite marks occur, in order of decreasing frequency (Becker et al., 1978). This chapter will discuss the treatment of minor orofacial injuries when airway obstruction or hypovolemic shock are not complicating factors. Because of their seriousness, these major injuries will usually be treated by emergency medical services.

Contusions and Ecchymoses

Contusions and ecchymoses are best treated with ice packs to accessible areas for the first 24 hours. This results in local vasoconstriction and minimizes the flow of blood to the traumatized area. In instances of extensive swelling, pressure dressings may be helpful. Later in the course of treatment application of warm packs helps resolve extravasated blood in the tissues. It is important to note that these lesions are often a diagnostic sign of possible underlying or related bony fractures. For example, a contusion in the floor of the mouth often signals a fracture of the mandible.

Abrasions

Treatment of abrasions primarily consists of careful cleansing of the wound. Gentle irrigation of the wound with warm water and soap helps to remove dirt and foreign material. The wound is then irrigated with copious amounts of normal saline and the surrounding skin is prepared with an antiseptic solution such as Betadine.[2] If foreign material still remains, cleansing with a brush and surgical soap may be required along with removal of specific individual debris with a sterile cotton tip, tissue forcep, or the tip of a no. 11 scalpel. Placement of a sterile dressing such as Xeroform[3] or Furacin[4] gauze over the wound will help in protecting the wound from further irritation and promoting healing. The dressing should be changed daily until the wound is healed.

Lacerations

It is essential to use local anesthesia in managing lacerations in children. When possible, regional block anesthesia should be used to avoid distortion of wounds. As with abrasions, one should be suspicious of foreign bodies within a wound. It is not uncommon for tooth fragments to be present. Appropriate soft tissue radiographs should be taken to rule out this possibility when the child sustains fractured teeth with lacerations.

Following wound debridement, as described above, the wound should be explored to delineate its anatomy and to assess any damage to nearby structures such as a parotid duct or gland, Wharton's duct, or a facial nerve. Only obviously nonviable tissue should be excised. It is best to use 5-0 or 6-0 nylon or silk sutures for skin suturing; 3-0 or 4-0 chromic gut sutures for repairing the musculature, such as the lip or tongue; and 4-0 or 5-0 plain gut sutures for mucosal closures. Suturing is done in layers, starting from the inside and moving to the outside. Interrupted suturing should be used, placing the sutures no farther than 2.5 millimeters apart. Nonresorbable sutures should be removed four days after

[2]Betadine Surgical Scrub, Purdue Frederick Co., Norwalk, Conn.
[3]Xeroform, Cheesebrough-Ponds Inc., Greenwich, Conn.
[4]Furacin Soluble Dressing, Eaton Laboratories, Norwich, N.Y.

placement. Dry wounds can be dressed with steri-strips and draining wounds can be covered with Xeroform gauze. The use of prophylactic antibiotics is recommended, with penicillin the drug of choice.

Punctures

Puncture wounds are treated similarly to lacerations. The wound must be cleansed, the damage assessed, and, if large enough, the puncture must be sutured in layers. Small punctures can be left to heal by secondary intention, especially in areas such as the palate.

Human Bite Marks

Human bite marks must be treated as serious injuries since devastating complications can result if proper treatment is not rendered. Frequently reported complications include recurrent infections, permanent joint stiffness, osteomyelitis and digital amputations. Less frequently occurring are extremity amputations, systemic sepsis, and death (Malinowski et al., 1979). Initially the wound should be cleansed, debrided if necessary, and left open. Administration of tetanus toxoid is recommended according to the previously described protocol. *Staphylococcus aureus* is the organism most frequently encountered in human bite wound infections, although other strains have been implicated (Goldstein et al., 1978; Malinowski et al., 1979). Antibiotics recommended include cephalosporin, penicillin, or clindamycin.

Minor bite wounds can be treated as traumatic ulcers with topical protectants such as Orabase.[5] A corticosteroid such as triamcinolene when added to the protectant (Kenalog in Orabase)[5] can help control resultant inflammation.

Avulsions

Avulsion injuries involve losses of portions of soft tissues. These can involve complex surgical procedures, and are best managed by oral and/or plastic surgeons. If a large segment of the skin has been lost, it should be located if possible for use in surgical repair.

Burns

Burns to the orofacial structure are not uncommon. They may be classified as electrical, thermal, or chemical.

The etiology, histologic, and clinical features of electrical burns have been well-reviewed (Needleman and Berkowitz, 1974). Minor electrical burns can be treated conservatively by repeated applications of topical antibiotics. They heal

[5]Orabase and Kenalog in Orabase, Squibb & Sons, Princeton, N.J.

with surprisingly little deformity. Tetanus toxoid should be administered if the patient is in need of a booster.

Major electrical burns require hospitalization because severe complications often occur. These include fluid loss, poor nutrition, and shock, as well as secondary hemorrhage from the labial arteries that may occur three to four days after injury. Careful daily debridement is necessary to remove necrotic tissue and stimulate the formation of healthy granulation tissue. Adhesive straps can be used for good approximation of wound edges and manipulation of muscle pull. Home care should include frequent saline rinses and massaging of burned tissue to increase blood supply.

Many burns require surgical repair, but the exact timing of the repair remains controversial. A delayed or conservative approach to the management of the acquired oral deformity is now recommended (Oeconomopoulos, 1962; Thomson et al., 1965; Fogh-Anderson and Sorensen, 1966; Pitts et al., 1969; Goldberg, 1969; Gifford et al., 1971; Ackerman and Goldfaden, 1971; Gormley et al., 1972). Several articles have been published recently recommending an intraoral acrylic splint with extraoral extensions be inserted soon after the trauma (Colcleugh and Ryan, 1976; Wright et al., 1977; Larson, 1977; Ryan, 1979). This appliance has proven successful in minimizing the contraction of the commissure, a long-term sequelae of electrical burns to the mouth.

Thermal burns involving small portions of the face should be covered with sterile dressings. The wound needs to be inspected every three or four days for healing progress and signs of infection. Antibiotics should be applied during the healing process, but greasy ointments should be avoided. Extensive second- or third-degree burns of the face are best referred to the hospital burn center.

Ulcerations of the oral mucosa that occur as results of thermal injuries usually heal uneventfully (McCarthy and Shklar, 1980). The ulcerative area should be kept covered with a thick paste. Topical steroids, such as triamcinolone, in an adhering paste (Kenalog in Orabase) can be helpful for healing and pain control. Complete healing of an ulcerative area caused by a thermal burn usually takes two to three weeks. Systemic analgesics can be helpful during the initial day or two following the injury.

Chemical agents accidentally or intentionally placed in the mouth result in severe and acute trauma to the oral mucosa (McGuigan, 1979). A white slough forms representing necrotic epithelium. As the slough is rubbed off, a bleeding, raw, and painful area is exposed. Caustic or corrosive burns of the mouth can result from ingesting liquid or solid (granules or powder) forms of alkalies or acids.

Symptoms from burns of the oral cavity occur immediately and range from minor discomfort to severe pain. Extensive burns, however, may destroy mucosal nerve endings and produce anesthesia. Excess salivation, drooling, and dysphagia occur due to irritation of oral and esophageal mucosa. Examination of the mouth may show edema, inflammation, and/or whitish areas. The presence of oral burns only documents exposure to a caustic agent and does not predict accurately the presence or absence of esophageal burns.

Immediate treatment consists of washing the caustic substance off the skin or mucosa with copious amounts of water. Neutralizing the caustic agent may produce heat and is no longer recommended.

Venereal Lesions

Gonorrhea

Most tissues of the oral cavity can be infected by the organism *Neisseira gonorrhoeae* (Chue, 1975). Most observers agree that the tonsils and oropharynx are the most frequent sites of involvement. The patient might or might not be symptomatic. The diagnosis of oral gonorrhea can be confirmed through culturing with a specialized medium, i.e., Thayer-Martin or Transgrow. The treatment is similar to that for genital gonorrhea (Emans and Goldstein, 1977). The following is a treatment regimen for oral gonorrhea:

Procaine penicillin G	100,000 μg/kg I.M.
and	
Probenecid (patients > 2 y)	25 mg/kg P.O. prior to I.M. penicillin
or	
Erythromycin (patients < 8 y)	40 mg/kg/day P.O. divided into 4 doses, × 7 days
or	
Tetracycline (patients > 8 y)	25 mg/kg P.O. STAT then 40–60 mg/kg/day divided into 4 doses, × 7 days

A follow-up culture should be taken several days after therapy.

Syphilis

When clinical examination indicates suspicion of syphilis, corroboration with serological tests is mandatory. Systemic antibiotic therapy is the treatment of choice for syphilis because of the offending organism *Treponema pallidum*'s sensitivity to the drug. Penicillin may be administered in the following schedule for primary or secondary syphilis or contact history:

Benzathine penicillin G	2.4 million μg I.M. (1.2 million μg I.M. in each buttock) (pediatric: 50,000 μg/kg)
or	
Procaine penicillin G	600,000 μg I.M. for 10 days (pediatric: 25,000–30,000 μg/kg)

Alternatives for the penicillin-allergic patient are erythromycin or tetracycline.

Herpes

Infection with the herpes simplex virus can be divided into two stages: the primary and secondary infections. In addition, two antigenically distinct subtypes exist: type 1, which generally accounts for nongenital infections, and type 2, which is responsible for genital lesions. They can be differentiated by culture and immunologic reactions. Type 2 oral lesions result from orogenital contact with a carrier (Chang et al., 1974). Management of type 1 and type 2 lesions is the same, although the type 2 virus is somewhat more virulent.

In most instances, clinical appearance of the primary or secondary form of herpetic stomatitis is diagnostic. Viral studies including culture and antibody demonstrations offer corroborative evidence.

The primary infection, i.e., acute herpetic gingivostomatitis, is a systemic disease and is currently treated only by supportive care. Bed rest, adequate fluid intake, and analgesics are essential. High-calorie foods, such as ice cream, chocolates, and milk shakes are well-tolerated, and provide adequate nutrition and fluid intake during the illness. Systemic analgesics and antipyretics, such as aspirin or acetaminophen, can reduce oral discomfort and help to control the elevated temperature. Topical anesthetic rinses can give temporary relief for the ulcerations. Due to their disagreeable tastes, many preparations, such as viscous Xylocaine[6] and Dyclonine (Dyclone),[7] are not accepted well by children. A mixture of Benadryl elixir[8] and Kaopectate[9] (1:1) is helpful and well-accepted.

No medication or formulations have proven curative for recurrent herpes labialis (ADA, 1979). Topical ether has been advocated to reduce the severity of and increase the intervals between episodes of infection (Pasruka et al., 1973). Lesions are treated symptomatically with topical bland emollient creams or ointments. When secondary infection is evident or likely, administration of topical antibiotics is recommended. A complete review of the current treatment of recurrent herpes simplex has been published (Tesini et al., 1977).

Genital Warts

Genital or venereal warts (Condyloma acuminatum) can occur on the lip, tongue, or hard palate. They are caused by a papovirus and are treated by excision with standard surgical techniques or electrocautery. Excision should include the base of the mucosa into which the pedicle or stalk inserts, to decrease the chance of recurrence.

[6]Xylocaine Viscous, Aster Pharmaceutical Products, Worcester, Mass.
[7]Dyclone solution, Dow Pharmaceutical, Indianapolis, Ind.
[8]Benadryl elixir, Parke-Davis & Co., Englewood, N.J.
[9]Kaopectate, Upjohn Company, Kalamazoo, Mich.

Injuries to the Dentition

Fractures

The mildest form of tooth fracture is the *infraction,* or *craze line*. This injury is readily evident by translumination, and requires no treatment. Follow-up is necessary to evaluate possible pulpal necrosis resulting from apecae trauma and pathosis.

Class I

The Class I fracture, or *fracture of the enamel only,* requires smoothing off of rough enamel edges. An acid-etch incisal-interproximal restoration often is unnecessary in these small fractures, since with wear both incisal edges usually become symmetrical. If cosmetics are a concern, the incisal edges may be adjusted with a diamond stone or disk to produce symmetry.

Class II

The Class II fracture, or *fracture of the enamel and dentin,* requires immediate protection. Exposed dentin should be lined with a calcium hydroxide preparation. One normally has the option of temporarily covering the enamel and dentin with either a partially built-up resin restoration or a stainless steel band. With suspicion of child abuse, however, follow-up care with completion of final restoration might be impossible. Therefore, the tooth should be restored with resin to its original size and shape using the acid-etch technique during the emergency visit.

Class III

Class III fractures involve the *pulp, enamel, and dentin*. If the exposure is small (< 1 mm) and apexification of the permanent tooth complete, direct pulp capping or partial pulpotomy (Cvek, 1978) with calcium hydroxide may be attempted. Although highly successful, these procedures require close follow-ups. Therefore, to decrease chances for failure and the need for careful follow-up, one might consider definitive one-stage pulp therapy such as pulpectomy and gutta-percha obturation for these pulpal exposures.

Definitive pulpectomy and obturation is the only treatment recommended for large or old pulpal exposures of teeth with complete apexification. If, however, the fracture exposes the pulp on an immature tooth with an open apex, a calcium hydroxide pulpotomy is the treatment of choice. This procedure will allow the apex to continue to develop, with definitive pulpal therapy becoming possible once the apex is complete. Restoration of the Class III fracture can be performed as soon as possible, even during the pulpal phase of treatment. The acid-etch resin restoration is usually adequate, although a post-core and crown may be needed if the coronal fracture is extensive.

Root

Root fractures sometimes occur, although less frequently than coronal fractures. Treatment consists of reduction and alignment of the fractured segments, if they are not adequately opposed. Placement of a splint to stabilize the coronal segment is required for two to four months. Splinting is ideally performed with resin, using the acid-etch technique. Healthy union of the fragments will occur with either cementum, dense connective tissue, or a periodontal-like tissue (Michanowicz et al., 1971). Antibiotic coverage with penicillin is recommended. Evidence of a developing radiolucency at the fracture site or apex requires pulpal obturation to that point. In most cases this treatment results in success. However, if the conventional pulpaltherapy does not result in resolution, an apicoectomy may be required.

Displacements

Subluxation

The mildest form of displacement injury is *subluxation,* or the loosening of the tooth in the alveolus without frank displacement. This injury requires no treatment except for dietary restrictions and good oral hygiene during the process of healing. Splinting is recommended only if the tooth is mobile to the point that normal function will result in continual aggravation of the injury. Close follow-up for possible pulpal necrosis is essential.

Extrusive Luxation

The *lateral or extrusive luxation* injury requires reduction of the displacement, under local anesthesia, with finger pressure. The involved tooth should be splinted for three weeks, during which time normal mobility patterns are reestablished. Antibiotic coverage and good oral hygiene is recommended to decrease the chance of bacteria extending down the periodontal ligament space and impeding healing. Follow-up is essential due to the high incidence of complications, such as pulpal necrosis (52%), pulpal obliteration (27%), progressive root resorption (11%), and loss of marginal bone support (10%) (Andreasen, 1970).

The mild to moderate intrusive luxation injury can be treated by allowing the tooth to reerupt spontaneously over a period of a few months. Orthodontic forces may help the tooth reestablish its normal relationship (Andreasen, 1977). Immediate repositioning should only be considered in a severe intrusion where the labial cortical plate has been severely compromised. With all intrusions, pulpal necrosis is almost certain and pulpal obturation is required.

Avulsion

The *avulsed or totally displaced tooth* must be reimplanted immediately. Delays dramatically decrease the prognosis for success. If the tooth is contaminated with debris, a gentle cleansing with normal saline should be performed prior to insertion. Once reimplanted, the tooth should be splinted for seven to 10 days (Andreasen, 1975a and 1975b). Beginning pulpal obturation in the hand before reimplantation results in loss of valuable time, increasing chances that the periodontal ligament will die. Damage to the periodontal ligament causes replacement external root resorption and possible root ankylosis. Pulp should be extirpated as soon as possible to decrease chances for inflammatory external root resorption to develop. Temporary obturation of the canal space should be performed with calcium hydroxide (Needleman, 1981a and 1981b). If the reimplantation shows no complications after one year, final obturation with gutta-percha should be performed.

Many of these principles for treatment of traumatized teeth apply to both permanent and primary teeth. However, there are some differences in philosophy and technique, a comprehensive discussion of which is presented elsewhere in the literature (Needleman, 1981a and 1981b) and should be reviewed.

Facial Bone Fractures

Facial fractures are relatively uncommon in children. They can occur during physical assault, however, with nasal fractures most frequent (45%), followed by mandibular fractures (32%), and zygomaticmaxillary complex and orbit fractures (20.5%) (Kaban et al., 1977).

Initial management of facial fractures requires attention to basic life-support means, such as airway maintenance, control of bleeding, and fluid management. Sedation of the young patient may be necessary to fully evaluate the fracture both clinically and radiographically. Temporary stabilization of the fracture is often helpful to control pain during acute stages. Proper bandaging (e.g., using Barton's bandage) of the facial bones can provide support and help to sedate the patient before he/she is transferred into the care of an oral surgeon.

Diagnosis of mandible fractures can usually be made by clinical examination. The fracture appears as an irregularity in the mandibular arch, with loss of proper dental occlusion, and occasionally with tears of the oral mucosa. Mandibular fractures most commonly occur in the bicuspid area. No active treatment is necessary if there are no signs of displacement. Often there is little discomfort with these injuries. Soft or liquid diet should be prescribed for four weeks, which allows time for sufficient union for the patient to eat normally. If displacement is evident and teeth are adjacent to the fracture site, interdental wire fixation can be undertaken. If no teeth are present, stabilization of mandibular fractures may be accomplished by open reduction.

Mandibular fractures can also occur in the subcondylar region. These often cause pain and tenderness in the region of the temporomandibular joint, as well as considerable trismus and displacement of the lower dental arch. Active treatment of these fractures is seldom necessary, but referral to an oral surgeon is mandatory for further evaluation and follow-up.

A comprehensive discussion of the definitive management of facial fractures is presented elsewhere in the literature (Sanders et al., 1979) and should be reviewed.

Appendix Sample form*

Instructions to Parents Concerning Head Injuries

Your examining physician considers it safe for your child to return home. Although your child has been thoroughly examined for evidence of head injury, certain signs of trouble may appear in the next 48 hours. Please observe your child carefully and telephone us should any of the following signs appear. Be sure your examining physician explains them to you and answers your questions before you leave the hospital.

Signs of Trouble

1. *Excessive drowsiness*

   Your child may well be exhausted by the ordeal surrounding the injury, but should be easily awakened by methods that you would ordinarily employ to awaken him from a deep sleep. If you cannot do this, notify the hospital.

2. *Persistent vomiting*

   Children will, in most cases, vomit one or more times following a severe head injury. Should the vomiting occur more than once or twice, or should it begin again hours after it has ceased, notify the hospital.

3. If one pupil appears to be larger than the other, notify the hospital.
4. If the child does not use either arm or leg as well as previously, or is unsteady in walking, notify the hospital.
5. Should speech become slurred or the child be apparently unable to talk, notify the hospital.
6. If severe headache occurs, particularly if it increases in severity and is not relieved by aspirin, notify the hospital.
7. Should the child complain of "seeing double" or should you detect any failure of the eyes to move together appropriately, notify the hospital.
8. Should a convulsion occur, place the child on one side and where he cannot fall, be sure there is ample room for him to breath, placing a firm object between the molar teeth to keep mouth open. Stay with the child until the convulsions begin to subside, and notify the hospital as soon as possible.

On the night following the head injury, or during any nap, it is advisable to awaken your child (every three hours) and look for any of these danger signs.

*Source: Emergency Room information sheet, The Children's Hospital Medical Center, Boston, Mass.

References

Ackerman, A.B. and Goldfaden, G.L.: Electrical Burns of the Mouth in Children. Arch. Dermat. 104:308, 1971.

American Academy of Pedodontics (AAP): Report of the Committee on Infectious Disease. (18th ed.). Chicago: AAP, 1977, p. 278.

American Dental Association (ADA): Accepted Dental Therapeutics. (38th ed.). Chicago: ADA, 1979, p. 286.

Andreasen, J.O.: Luxation of Permanent Teeth Due to Trauma. Scand. J. Dent. Res. 78:273, 1970.

Andreasen, J.O.: The Effect of Splinting Upon Periodontal Healing after Reimplantation of Permanent Incisors in Monkeys. Acta. Odont. Scand. 33:313, 1975a.

Andreasen, J.O.: Periodontal Healing after Reimplantation of Traumatically Avulsed Human Teeth. Acta. Odont. Scand. 33:325, 1975b.

Andreasen, J.O.: Examination and Diagnosis of Traumatic Injuries. Paper presented at the 30th Annual Meeting of the American Academy of Pedodontics, Miami Beach, 1977.

Becker, D.B.; Needleman, H.L.; and Kotelchuck, M.: Child Abuse and Dentistry: Orofacial Trauma and its Recognition by Dentists. J. Am. Dent. Assoc. 97:24, 1978.

Chang, T.; Fiumara, N.J.; and Weinstein, L.: Genital Herpes: Some Clinical and Laboratory Observations. J. Am. Med. Assoc. p. 544, 1974.

Chue, P.W.Y.: Gonorrhea—Its Natural History, Oral Manifestations, Diagnosis, Treatment and Prevention. J. Am. Dent. Assoc. 90:1297, 1975.

Colcleugh, R.L. and Ryan, J.E.: Splinting Electrical Burns of the Mouth in Children. Plast. Reconstr. Surg. 58:239, 1976.

Craig, J.W. and Hargreaves, J.A.: Assessment of Injury with Aims and Principles of Treatment. In Hargreaves, J.A.; Craig, J.W.; and Needleman, H.L. (ed.) The Management of Traumatized Anterior Teeth of Children. (2nd ed.). Edinburgh: Livingstone, 1981, p. 10.

Cvek, N.: A Clinical Report on Partial Pulpotomy and Capping with Calcium Hydroxide in Permanent Incisors with Complicated Crown Fractures. J. Endod. 4:232, 1978.

Emans, S.J. and Goldstein, D.P.: Venereal Disease. In Pediatric and Adolescent Hygecology. (1st ed.). Boston: Little, Brown & Co., 1977, p. 113.

Fogh-Anderson, P. and Sorensen, B.: Electric Mouth Burns in Children, Treatment and Prevention. Acta. Chir. Scand. 131:214, 1966.

Gifford, G.H.; Marty, A.T.; and MacCollum, D.W.: The Management of Electrical Mouth Burns in Children. Pediatrics 47:113, 1971.

Goldberg, M.H.: Electrical Trauma to the Oral Cavity. J. Oral Surg. 27:190, 1969.

Goldstein, E.J.; Citron, D.M.; Wield, B.; Blackman, U.; Sutter, V.L.; Miller, T.A.; and Finegold, S.M.: Bacteriology of Human and Animal Bite Wounds. J. Clin. Microbiol. 8:667, 1978.

Gormley, M.B.; Marshall, J.; Jarrett, W.; and Bromberg, B.: Thermal Trauma: A Review of 22 Electrical Burns of the Lip. J. Oral Surg. 30:531, 1972.

Kaban, L.B.; Mulliken, J.B.; and Murray, J.E.: Facial Fractures in Children. Plast. Reconstr. Surg. 59:15, 1977.

Larson, T.H.: Splinting Oral Electrical Burns in Children, Report of Two Cases. J. Dent. Child. 44:383, 1977.

Malinowski, R.W.; Strate, R.G.; Perry, J.F.; and Fischer, R.P.: Management of Human Bite Injuries of the Hand. J. Trauma 19:655, 1979.

McCarthy, P.L. and Shklar, G.: Traumatic Lesions of Oral Mucosa. In Diseases of the Oral Mucosa. (2nd ed.). Philadelphia: Lea and Febiger, 1980, p. 334.

McGuigan, M.A.: Caustics. Clin. Toxic Rev. 1:12, 1979.

Michanowicz, A.E.; Michanowicz, J.P.; and Abou-Rass, M.: Cementogenic Repair of Root Fractures. J. Am. Dent. Assoc. 88:569, 1971.

Needleman, H.L.: Injuries to Deciduous Teeth. In Hargreaves, J.A.; Craig, J.W.; and Needleman, H.L. (ed.). The Management of Traumatized Anterior Teeth of Children. (2nd ed.). Edinburgh: Livingstone, 1981a, p. 142.

Needleman, H.L.: Total Tooth Displacement and Reimplantation. In Hargreaves, J.A.; Craig, J.W.; and Needleman, H.L. (ed.). The Management of Traumatized Anterior Teeth of Children. (2nd ed.). Edinburgh: Livingstone, 1981b, p. 98.

Needleman, H.L. and Berkowitz, R.J.: Electric Trauma to the Oral Tissues in Children. J. Dent. Child. 41:19, 1974.

Oeconomopoulos, C.T.: Electrical Burns in Infancy and Early Childhood. Am. J. Dis. Child. 103:67, 1962.

Pasruka, J.S.; Nayizar, K.C.; and Pasruka, A.: A New Method for Treatment of Herpes Simplex. Arch. Dermat. 107:775, 1973.

Pitts, W.; Pickrell, K.; Quinn, G.; and Massengill, R.: Electrical Burns of Lips and Mouths in Infants and Children. Plast. Reconstr. Surg. 44:471, 1969.

Ryan, J.E.: Prosthetic Treatment of Electrical Burns to the Oral Cavity. J. Prosthet. Dent. 42:434, 1979.
Sanders, B.; Brady, F.A.; and Johnson, R.: Injuries. In Sanders, B. Pediatric Oral and Maxillofacial Surgery. (1st ed.). St. Louis: C.V. Mosby, 1979, p. 330.
Tesini, D.; Chang, T.; Ficarelli, J.; and Kane, J.: Recurrent Herpes Simplex Virus Infection. Part II, Treatment and Pathogenesis. J. Pedodont. 1:208, 1977.
Thomson, H.G.; Juckes, A.M.; and Famer, A.M.: Electrical Burns to the Mouth of Children. Plast. Reconstr. Surg. 35:466, 1965.
Wright, G.Z.; Colcleugh, R.L.; and Davidge, L.K.: Electric Burns to the Commisures of the Lips. J. Dent. Child. 44:377, 1977.

Chapter 9

Interviewing, Child Protection, and Reporting Protocol

Edward J. Goldson

Introduction

One of the most difficult tasks the practitioner has to perform is interviewing parents suspected of abusing their children. Although awareness of child abuse has increased dramatically, when confronted with the issue the practitioner is often unprepared for the events that transpire. There is a tendency to avoid what can be, and often is, a very unpleasant and stressful situation. This is particularly true for the office-based, fee-charging practitioner.

Child abuse in all of its manifestations—nonaccidental trauma, neglect/failure to thrive, and sexual abuse—are all realities in our health care delivery system. It is important for the practitioner, therefore, to have interviewing skills and a knowledge of immediate child protection and abuse reporting procedures to effectively deal with such problems that might occur in his/her dental practice. This chapter will discuss an approach to interviewing persons suspected of abusing children, protective services for those children, and a reporting protocol.

Interviewing

Reluctance

Despite overwhelming evidence to the contrary, many people still believe that it is only the poor or psychologically deranged who abuse their children. This is not the case. Abuse occurs in all segments of our society, and our perception of the abuser and our reluctance or discomfort in relating to him/her and to the abused child must be evaluated with this in mind.

Practitioners in health care institutions delivering episodic primary care to children who often come from a different socioeconomic class than their own might find it easier to deal with abusive parents. However, the practitioner must accept the fact that child abuse occurs across all ethnic and socioeconomic boundaries and that it will and does occur in the middle class that seeks office-based care. When suspected child abuse occurs in ethnic and/or socioeconomic groups similar to his/her own, the private practitioner may feel very uncomfortable in pursuing and identifying the problem. The interview often will be difficult as a result.

Initially the practitioner may deny that abuse has occurred, or disbelieve that this could be happening to people who are ethnically or socioeconomically similar to the practitioner. Nevertheless, as health practitioners we must deal with these issues as objectively and compassionately as possible.

Child abuse is a medical-social-psychological disorder and, therefore, one of many problems that health practitioners must confront. There are many experiences in medicine and dentistry that are exceedingly distasteful. If a physician establishes the diagnosis of leukemia, he/she does the patient and family a gross disservice if the physician does not relate this information to them and provide therapy, support, and guidance. If a dentist diagnoses a serious dental condition whose treatment will be uncomfortable, lengthy, and expensive, certainly similar avoidance would be a disservice. Avoidance of such an unpleasant task is practicing less than optimal health care. If the health practitioner avoids dealing with the issue of child abuse when it presents itself, he/she is doing the patient and family a disservice and, indeed, may allow for future injury. Child abuse is a health issue that must be appropriately diagnosed and treated.

Some physicians and dentists are more comfortable than others with dealing with child abuse. Arguments have been raised by physicians and dentists questioning the merits of reporting suspected abuse. One argument is that parents have the prerogative to deal with their child as they choose, another that it is not the practitioner's duty or business to report child abuse. Other arguments assume that if the practitioner alienates the parents, he/she will no longer be able to help the child.

As health professionals we have a responsibility and mandate, under law, to report to the appropriate authorities any case in which there is reasonable cause to suspect that child abuse and/or neglect is occurring or has occurred. Every state in the United States has a child abuse reporting act.

In addition to being legally required, reporting also initiates a series of interventions that can be of enormous aid to the family and which might serve to protect the child from further injury. Evidence suggests that abusive families who were reported and were required by court order to attend parenting classes were better able to deal with the problem of abuse than were parents who refused or voluntarily began participation in parenting classes. Furthermore, those parents who started on a purely voluntary basis dropped out of the program more frequently.

There is evidence to suggest that although the task of reporting or even investigating abuse is distasteful, when it is done with sensitivity and in as nonjudgmental a manner as possible, the health practitioner does not lose the patient from his/her practice. The practitioner may even be able to solidify and enhance the relationship with the family. The abuse may, indeed, be a cry for help. Consider this as an approach toward the complicated dynamics of child abuse, rather than the stance so frequently taken that the abuse merely reflects a bad parent who has lashed out at his/her child or has willfully neglected the child. When the more positive approach is taken parents frequently are not alienated and the practitioner is able to continue as a significant support to both the child and the family.

Courses of Action

The first course that the health practitioner can take in the office when he/she suspects child abuse is filing a report. By doing so the practitioner is not accusing or convicting a parent. It is a call for help, asking for the delivery of services to a family. Using the medical model and making the assumption that abuse is, among other things, a medical problem, the report can be viewed as a consultation with or a turning toward another expert for help dealing with a sensitive and difficult problem.

An alternative course, not reporting, is unacceptable from moral, ethical, and legal viewpoints.

A third course is to wait and see what happens. "Maybe the abuse was a one-time crazy accident." When the health practitioner indulges in this kind of thinking and waits, it becomes more and more difficult to deal with the situation. The health practitioner can become involved in a dangerous situation. Believing that the problem will subside and end in time is a fallacy.

The Interview and Responses

The task in interviewing a parent suspected of abuse is not to diagnose abuse. The health practitioner is not expected to be a detective. The responsibility is to identify the difficulty, alert the parents to the concerns, and notify the appropriate authorities so that they can pursue the problem. The health practitioner is not an inquisitor. He/she is seeking information about the well-being of a patient, and this is the attitude with which the interview should be conducted.

First, it is important that the health practitioner be aware of how he/she views the problem, the symptoms, and his/her role. It becomes easier when the health practitioner views child abuse from a relatively dispassionate standpoint as a medical issue. True, one's initial response may be revulsion. However, these feelings should be superseded by a desire to help and by the assumption of a supportive stance.

Psychological and other professional responses should be similar to those for other serious injuries or conditions that might have grave implications for the patient and family. The health professional can perhaps more objectively determine what symptoms mean when he/she can go beyond the revulsion. If nonaccidental trauma or neglect are seen as cries for help and expressions of psychological and social dysfunction, and if the health practitioner is trained not to disregard child abuse but to confront it, it is easier for the practitioner to assume a supportive and understanding role irregardless of his/her revulsion. The health practitioner should not assume a judgmental or accusatory attitude, but one that is helpful and responsive.

Once a constructive attitude has been established, the next step is to identify how any existing injuries or lesions occurred. It is reasonable to be direct in asking questions, but at the same time it is important to use tact and sensitivity to the responses. Nonverbal cues and nuances should also be noted.

The quest for information is acceptable and few parents will deny that information. However, when what is heard and what is known about children does not coincide with what is known about possible causes of the injury or lesion evaluated, the task to probe further is paramount. One guiding principle is that certain injuries are age-appropriate. As discussed in Chapters 3 through 6, when the injury or lesion does not match what is known about the child and the child's maturity both physically and cognitively, then abuse or neglect must be suspected. If it is concluded that an injury or lesion could not have been accidental, the health practitioner must relate this concern to the parent. This can be done in the following manner:

> Mrs. Jones, I hear and understand what you have said about how Johnny injured his tooth, yet I have difficulty with this. From what I have seen in the past and what I know about children, this could not have occurred in a purely accidental manner. Can you give me any more information?

The parent will probably recognize very quickly what has been said and have any one of several responses.

One of the first responses will be *anger:* "How dare you imply that I. . . ." or "Do you think I would. . . ." The health practitioner could be put on the defensive by this response unless he/she recognizes that the parent is in psychological pain. An appropriate counter-response could be: "No, I am not accusing you of . . . I know that you love your child and that you would not consciously hurt . . . but I am concerned about this injury." This does not skirt the issue; indeed, it may establish a level of trust. Very often the parent's response will be to test you. The unspoken question may be: "Are you my friend or my enemy?" or "Can I trust you?" The health professional should be firm and professional yet compassionate and supportive. This can be accomplished even during a rather direct interview.

As the interview is conducted, it is important to recognize that the parent often needs attention. Focus should not be entirely on the child and the parent's call for help negated or ignored. Many parents who actively abuse or neglect their children are themselves childlike. Therefore, the interviewer may be cast into the role of mature, responsible adult. Many abusive parents are overwhelmed when the health professional recognizes that parenting is difficult. This can be one of the greatest links in the therapeutic alliance. Demonstration that the health practitioner will not abandon them but will support them as they go through this difficult time is essential to this alliance.

Another response might be *denial:* "I don't know what you are talking about" or "I had nothing to do with this and I am just telling you what Jimmy told me." A response might also be very *detached,* such as: "Oh, that's interesting. Could you show me what you mean?" or "This is very intriguing."

Depression can be reflected in parental response: "Oh, I don't know how this happened. This child is so difficult and active and I don't know how to manage him. I get so tired trying to deal with all of the things that are going on at home." This response may lead to tears and occasionally an admission such as: "Yes, I did hit him but I really didn't mean to and I didn't realize I had hit him so hard." There are obviously a number of other responses that could take place, but these represent the most common in the spectrum.

Child Protection and Reporting

In any of the circumstances described above the health practitioner does not have to accuse the parent. He/she can matter-of-factly express concern with the injury or lesion and recognition that parents desire to do the best for their child. It is the professional and legal obligation of the practitioner, however, to make the appropriate authorities aware of his/her suspicion. The practitioner should describe what will be done and explain why, and then should file the report as prescribed in state law. This usually means a verbal report to the department of social services and/or the police. At the time of the call, which hopefully can be made in the parent's presence, the dentist should be prepared to state his concern or reasons for suspecting abuse (physical findings, etc.). He/she should also be prepared to provide the names and addresses of the involved parties. Some commitment should be obtained from the referral agency as to what the plan of action will be, who will contact the parents, and when that contact will take place. It should be indicated whether immediate child protection is necessary and what services will be provided.

Ramifications might result from reporting. These can include anger and threats. However, many parents are relieved that a concern has been honestly raised. Although they may deny having inflicted the injury, they are often secretly relieved that someone is concerned, helping, and showing them they will not be abandoned. The way the interview is conducted, the expression of concern, and the offer of continued help and support all will make a difference in the outcome.

The health practitioner who is not intimidated by anger or tears demonstrates mature concern that most parents will respond to. Never forget that parents who injure their children, for whatever reasons, are themselves in pain and need help. By raising the issue of abuse honestly, the dentist recognizes distress and responds to needs. This often protects parents and their children from more injury and pain, a most desirable result.

Summary

Health practitioners must be aware of the incidences of child abuse and neglect in all classes of society, and recognize general reluctance in diagnosing them as causes of injuries and lesions. When confronted with suspected child abuse and neglect, the health practitioner must be competent to conduct an interview attentive to the situation. Moral, professional, and legal obligations demand immediate child protection and reporting in cases of abuse or neglect.

References

Goldson, E.: Child Abuse: A Social-Psychological-Medical Disorder. In Gellert, E. Psychosocial Aspects of Pediatric Care. New York: Grune and Stratton Inc., 1978.

Helfer, R.E. and Kempe, C.H.: The Battered Child. (2nd ed.). Chicago: University of Chicago Press, 1974.

Helfer, R.E. and Kempe, C.H.: Child Abuse and Neglect: The Family and the Community. Cambridge, Mass.: Ballinger, 1976.

Kempe, C.H. and Helfer, R.D.: Helping the Battered Child and his Family. Philadelphia: J.B. Lippincott, 1972.

Sanders, R. and Wymand, M.D.: Resistance to Dealing with Parents of Battered Children. Pediatrics 50:853, 1972.

Wolfe, D.A.; Aragona, J.; Kaufman, K.; and Sandler, J.: The Importance of Adjudication in the Treatment of Child Abusers: Some Preliminary Findings. Child Abuse and Neglect 4:1, 1980.

Chapter 10

Child Protection Teams

Candace A. Grosz and JoAnn Avila

Introduction

The increased emphasis placed on training programs and community awareness in the field of child protective services has paralleled the increased reporting of child abuse and neglect cases. In attempting to understand and treat numerous cases of child abuse, professionals have become overwhelmed with the complexities of the family services and the management of mounting caseloads. This prompted Dr. C.H. Kempe and Ms. B. Elmer and H. Boardman to devise an effective and efficient method for diagnosing and treating child abuse in a coordinated manner. Their efforts resulted in the establishment of the first child protection team in the late 1950s (Kempe, 1976). These hospital-based teams consisted of a pediatrician, social worker, and nurse. Later teams expanded to include local community agencies and were called community-based teams. While there are a number of different names by which teams are known, perhaps the most common are child protection teams, child advocacy teams, and multidisciplinary review teams.

Legal Role

Child protection teams are usually established in each county to report cases of child abuse or neglect. These teams are considered mandatory if they operate within specific guidelines outlined in Article 10 of the 1977 Child Protection Act. Voluntary teams need not follow the guidelines of the act. Voluntary teams also do not have the legal authority that the mandatory teams do to effect different plans of action if they disagree with dispositions reached by local social services agencies.

Team Composition

Although an ideal team should have five or six members, each team should have no fewer than three members, commonly referred to as the "nuclear team" (Schmitt, 1976). Nuclear team members are usually professionals who have had direct involvement with the family. The other team members' participation is consultative. They are referred to as the "consultative team" (Schmitt, 1976). When possible, the team should consist of:

- Pediatrician
- Attorney
- Social worker
- Representative of a local law enforcement agency
- Representative of a public health department (nurse)
- Representative of a public school district
- Representative of the lay community
- In an area with a significant racial or ethnic minority, a representative of that minority should serve as a lay member.

Certainly the professional(s) who were directly involved in the treatment and evaluation of the case under discussion should be present at team meetings.

To facilitate organization and distribution of case material, it is essential to designate a team coordinator. This person usually directs the meeting, records the suggestions and recommendations discussed, and communicates that information to the appropriate agencies.

It is not appropriate, and often is counter-productive, to allow family members to be present during discussion of their own case, although recommendations are fully shared following the meeting via a social service or other family worker.

Team Function

The team's function will vary depending on the size of the community it serves and the organization to which it is linked. Two of the teams most commonly referred to are the community-based (urban or rural) and the hospital-based.

A community-based child protection team is generally established to serve a specific geographical area, such as a county or city, and the cases they review are usually confined to referrals made on families who are residents of the community. In an urban setting, the role of the team is likely to include a consultative function, simply because of the greater availability of expert advice in the field of child advocacy.

The teams based in small or private hospitals generally restrict their reviews to cases that are being or have been followed in the hospital. Hospital-based teams draw their core membership from within their own institution; however, it is critical that the county social service worker, county health department nurse, and other professionals directly involved with the family be present at the meeting. Every effort should be made to invite and include them in the review, especially if the team will be making diagnostic and treatment decisions. In state university hospitals, the consultative and direct evaluation roles are combined. Often these teams are good resources for unusual or difficult cases.

Conducting an effective and efficient child protection team meeting is a major challenge. There are many issues that can block the desired function, development of a family treatment plan. These plans are complex and multifaceted, and in the normal course of evaluation much detailed information is gathered by each discipline. Common dilemmas at team conferences include: dwelling on one problem or one family member, relating long anecdotes, using team time for ventilation, or planning community programs. Therefore, child protection teams have adapted the problem-oriented approach as a means of integrating and condensing this volume of information while giving direction to both child protection team discussion and treatment planning (Schmitt et al., 1976).

Problem-Oriented Approach

A tentative problem-oriented record is drawn up prior to the team conference. It outlines major problems for all family members rather than an individual patient, and encompasses all disciplines, including medical, psychosocial, and legal. Tentative recommendations are included where possible, with focuses on outlining gaps in information and prioritizing needs. Two or three primary questions that the team must address are spelled out. Usually, these focus on prognosis for treatment, custody and placement of children, and use of juvenile or criminal court. A set of operational rules for team meetings have evolved with use of this problem-oriented approach. This helps the team stay focused and productive within the ever-present time constraints.

Dynamics of Interaction

There are four dynamics of interaction that address team output in child abuse and neglect management. When these dynamics function within a team framework, they can be managed constructively and demonstrate major benefits of the multidisciplinary team approach.

First, there is the simple need to coordinate numerous public and private services for the family. A team approach decreases confusion for family members and workers and helps reduce duplication or serious gaps. As more and more social services are deleted with budgetary restraints, such maximum use of limited resources becomes even more crucial.

Second, the services to a typical abusive family require many professional disciplines, each with its unique perspective of cause and effective remedy. Medicine, law, and psychotherapy are three of the major disciplinary frameworks in this field. Without a team, work may proceed with contradictory goals. Team members have the opportunities to articulate similarities and differences, choose the most appropriate method, and change approaches if ineffectiveness occurs. They can essentially tailor the treatment plan with the broadest possible data base in a complementary, rather than conflicting manner. Efficient use of all disciplines is increased through role clarification. A unified professional view can be presented to the family and the courts after a consensus is reached in team discussion. When a consensus is not possible, several recommendations can be made in an orderly manner.

Third, there is a tendency for persons to identify with either the parent or the child of an abusive family, so that any one professional will find it difficult to have a comprehensive, objective view of what is needed. Often successful treatment requires many social service workers, with some clearly identified to serve the parent and others to serve the child. The team offers a wide view since some members are not directly involved with the family. These consultants are often more able to judge whether or not progress is being made. The increased visibility regarding performance may be uncomfortable for some individual practitioners; however, the increased protection for the interest of the child and parents makes it worthwhile.

Fourth, the team provides a forum to share decision-making and move toward greater community responsibility for the problems of child abuse and neglect. This can extend to sharing the responsibility of program development and professional and public education through a child protection council. No one agency or professional can adequately address the needs of abusive families. However, "turfism," where social service workers feel protective, possessive, and threatened by involvement of others in the affairs of "their" families, is not uncommon.

Confidentiality

Confidentiality can be cited as a reason why information and decisions cannot be shared. Certainly, there are legal considerations making establishment of safeguards necessary to protect families' privacy. However, too often confidentiality is used as a smoke screen when professionals and agencies are unwilling to trust and share, even though families may benefit significantly through more comprehensive and competent services.

Cohesion

As the child protection team becomes a more cohesive group, it is easier to share decisions. The team can be a major support at times when treatment fails and a child is reinjured, when termination of parental rights is recommended, or in cases of serious risk to newborns when intervention can mean the difference between life or death. The team can also help persons cope with the feelings of anger, frustration, and disbelief that surface frequently in child abuse and neglect. In these ways, a multidisciplinary approach works to decrease the emotional drain for all disciplines and the high burnout rate of social service workers.

Private practitioners may find it difficult to strike the desired balance in team participation. Team members may seem to take over the case to such an extent that the referring physician feels eliminated. To prevent this, continue to inquire regarding results of evaluation and recommendations, and ask for a copy of any written team summary. Try to attend the team meeting and outline the needs you see for the family as well as services you can provide or arrange. Too often, good intentions to provide feedback to referring persons do not materialize and may need to be pursued.

At times the private practitioner may be relieved to turn this demanding situation over to the team and withdraw. When this happens, the team and especially the family loses a valuable asset. Often, the referring person has known the family for a long time, can provide a perspective very different from social services and police evaluations done during the crisis of reporting, and offers a badly needed resource for continuity of care.

Review Process

When a child protection team is requested to review a case, there are a number of evaluations to consolidate. Coordination of professional assistance is imperative, and it should be made clear to each individual the kind of involvement that will be expected of them during this process.

The team needs as much factual information as possible. Explicit descriptions of physical injuries, child's developmental status, parent-child interaction, social histories of each parent, etc., all need to be considered by the child protection team at the time of referral and at every point thereafter when treatment is being planned.

Professionals sometimes believe they must know all of the facts before they contact protective services or a child protection team about a child's care. Although it is up to the experienced professional treating a suspicious case to evaluate the need for intervention, any information used in his diagnosis of abuse that is provided to the Child Protection team could be of significant importance in assessing safety of the home. Depending upon the professional's knowledge of or association with the child/family, he/she should be prepared to offer recommendations or suggestions when treatment is being planned.

Assisting the Professional

While the child protection team expects input from the reporting professional, there are also a number of functions a child protection team can perform to assist the professional. These include:

- Receive reports of suspected abuse and/or neglect
- Make a diagnostic assessment
- Perform crisis intervention whenever necessary
- Develop an immediate plan to protect the child
- Develop recommendations for long-term therapy

Using the team for consultative purposes is another way to obtain assistance, not only in the diagnosis and treatment of child abuse and neglect cases, but also in helping to decide if a case is at a preventative stage or at a reportable level. Overall, the use of child protection teams has become an increasingly valuable method for reviewing cases concerning children at risk. In addition, teams have been instrumental in providing supportive, consultative, and resource services, not only for the family, but also for the primary care practitioner. Consequently, more child protection teams are being established.

Although not all hospitals or counties have child protection teams, there are several ways to find out if one exists in a community:

- Contact the director of the department of social services in that county.

- Consult with the child welfare division of the department of social services in that county.
- Contact the Regional Resource Center of the U.S. Department of Health and Human Services.

Summary

The use of a multidisciplinary review team may be mandatory or voluntary. Benefits include information sharing, completeness of data collection, enlarging family perspectives, shared decision making, and a consolidated and coordinated case plan for treatment of parents and children. Team structure, legal authority and responsibility, and use of a problem-oriented approach are paramount for efficiency.

References

Helfer, R. and Schmidt, R.: The Community-based Child Abuse and Neglect Program. In Helfer, R. and Kempe, C.H. (ed.) Child Abuse and Neglect: The Family and the Community. Cambridge, Mass.: Ballinger, 1976, p. 232.

Kempe, C.H.: Forward. In Schmitt, B.D. (ed.) The Child Protection Team Handbook: A Multidisciplinary Approach to Managing Child Abuse and Neglect. New York: Garland, 1976.

Schmitt, B.C. (ed.): The Child Protection Team Handbook: A Multidisciplinary Approach to Managing Child Abuse and Neglect. New York: Garland, 1976, p. 9.

Schmitt, B.D.; Grosz, C.A.; and Carroll, C.A.: The Child Protection Team: A Problem-Oriented Approach. In Helfer, R.E. and Kempe, C.H. (ed.) Child Abuse and Neglect: The Family and the Community. Cambridge, Mass.: Ballinger, 1976.

Chapter 11

Legal Aspects of Child Abuse

Donald C. Bross

Introduction

Substantiated reports of child abuse and neglect are sufficiently numerous (NCCAN, 1981) that every dental professional can expect to treat patients who are abused or neglected. Any failure on the part of the dental practitioner to be aware of his/her professional and legal duties and protections in this area must concern both the individuals and the profession as a whole (Becker et al., 1978).

Increased recognition of abuse and neglect has brought rapid changes within arms of the legal system and medical, dental, and social services. Among the most important developments are impositions of new legal duties on medical and dental professionals and the growing impacts of these professions on the legal presentations of child abuse and neglect cases. These legal developments and their implications for dental professionals will be discussed in this chapter. The professional's role as witness will be addressed in the following chapter.

Basic knowledge of the legal concepts and practices pertaining to child protection is paramount. Definitions of child abuse and neglect must be understood in relative detail to show that legal definitions are generally the product of many factors, including scientific or professional knowledge and community values. The various ways in which malpractice liability has been assessed, and may be assessed in the future, must be examined with the goals of improving professional practice and lowering risks of recovery against the dental professional. The dental professional has been enabled, with protection, to act in a measured way to improve the situation of an abused child and the family. Reassurance about his/her role in reporting a case can be found in several specific legal protections and must be reviewed as not only another aspect of malpractice issues, but also as a useful introduction to the dental professional's role as child advocate.

Several aspects of the legal perspective of child abuse and neglect give the dental professional acting in this type of case an understanding of his/her responsibilities, liabilities, protections, and powers. The idea of health professionals being required to serve the public's health as well as that of the individual patient is not entirely new, nor is the idea of legally mandating protection of children. The union of these two traditions in the current legal system for child protection is, however, a recent development. The differences between the criminal and civil responses to cases of child abuse and neglect should be understood.

Privacy Interests, Public Health, and *parens patriae*

Most societies are premised constitutionally on great deference to private interest. In the areas of family life and sexual matters (*Meyer v. Nebraska,* 1923; *Pierce v. Society of the Sisters,* 1925; *Griswold v. Connecticut,* 1965), parents universally are presumed to know what is best for their children and to have the power to enforce what they believe is best. For the greatest majority of children and families, these rights are observed without challenge, because there is rarely reason to question the presumption that children are being raised reasonably, if imperfectly. As the extent to which some children have not been minimally cared for has become better documented, cases in which the presumption in favor of parents could not be left unchallenged have forced the attention of health care providers, the courts, and the public. The presumption in favor of family privacy and integrity persists but can be overcome whenever a child's life or health is in danger.

In a similar fashion, recognition of a right to keep communications to treating professionals confidential has been recognized as a general rule by court decisions and legislation (Paulsen, 1974), even though exceptions have increased (*Tarasoff v. Regents of the University of California,* 1976; *Landeros v. Flood,* 1976). Notwithstanding a desirable emphasis on individual privacy, the demands of public health have selectively overridden rights of privacy for many years. By 1917, some 38 communicable diseases were officially reportable in the United States (Gordon, 1965), primarily to control epidemics that the doctor-patient private arrangement could not guard against. The confidential relationship between health care provider and patient, even for such stigmatized conditions as venereal disease, was overridden to protect a larger group of potential patients. And early in this century, the U.S. Supreme Court ruled that immunizations could be compelled over an individual's objection to vaccination (*Jacobson v. Massachusetts,* 1905). For disease reporting and mass immunizations, the "class" to be protected consists of most of the public or, in effect, all of those not immune from a specific disease.

A separate doctrine, *parens patriae,* is also important in understanding laws developed to protect children. The doctrine evolved from earlier principles that the king or state could act as father on behalf of incompetents within the realm. Rather than being directed at the protection of children as a class, it allows a court to put itself "in the position of a wise, affectionate and careful parent, and make provision for the (particular) child accordingly" (*Finlay v. Finlay,* 1925).

These legal principles and traditions are the foundation for child abuse reporting laws that first became effective in a remarkably short period, from 1963 to 1966, in all 50 states (Paulsen, 1966). The role of the health care provider in reporting suspected abuse and neglect can now be reviewed extensively.

A Protected Class

Statutory recognition of children as a group unable to protect itself from misuse began as early as 1802 in England with the first child labor law (Robertson, 1974).

Early efforts to protect children from harsh effects of industrialization, to protect children and others from epidemics, and to assure mass educational opportunity, generally bypassed the issue of maltreatment at the hands of caretakers. The case of Mary Ellen in the 1970s marks the first significant legal recognition of abuse at home in the United States (Fontana, 1964).

United States Supreme Court decisions are a measure of the more rapid development now occurring with respect to children's legal rights. Until 1944 in *Prince v. Massachusetts,* and again in 1967 in the *In re Gault* case, the Supreme Court had not ruled that the Constitution contains guarantees for children other than those derivative from rights held by their parents. During the ensuing years, numerous cases on illegitimacy, termination of the parent-child legal relationship, mental health commitments, and other issues have marked a great increase in litigation on behalf of children throughout the American legal system. The importance of these cases for the health care professional is obvious: individuals charged with duties to care for or protect children will be increasingly held accountable for their actions.

Criminal and Civil ''Prosecution''

A person who injures a child may be criminally prosecuted, much as any perpetrator is prosecuted for such crimes as battery, assault, rape, or murder. The police are, of course, the primary agency involved in criminal investigations. Criminal laws exist principally to punish and deter perpetrators, with initiation and further processing of the prosecution carried out by an independent governmental prosecutor such as a district or state's attorney. For a conviction to occur and be upheld proof must be beyond a reasonable doubt and numerous restrictions on search and seizure, self-incrimination and representation by an attorney must be satisfied.

While in some cases of child abuse and neglect the untreatability of the defendant or severity of the offense strongly indicates prosecution, in most cases civil adjudication of the matter is easier and provides more alternatives for appropriate legal intervention in a family. Even in the worst cases of abuse and neglect, assuming the children survive, civil adjudication should take place simultaneously with criminal prosecution to assure the long-term safety of the children by freeing them for adoption or by a comparable long-term resolution.

In contrast with criminal prosecutions, the civil remedies of foster care, treatment for the child and parents, protection of the child's property rights, appointment of a long-term guardian ad litem, or permanent placement with a safe family, can occur by demonstrating that, at least, it is more likely than not or, at most, there is clear and convincing evidence that the child has been abused or neglected and that one or more of these remedies is needed. The civil process rarely results in a parent's imprisonment, since that is not the purpose of a civil action. Rather, the purpose of a ''dependency or neglect'' action is to determine whether there must be some intervention, therapeutic if possible, in the child's life in order to assure his/her safety and well-being. The primary agency for civil investigations and treatment of child abuse and neglect in most American counties is the protective services division of the local social services department.

The power of the civil approach is that it is more clearly directed to improving the child's situation; treats the parents in a noncriminal and, therefore, less stigmatizing fashion; and requires lesser evidentiary standards but can, nevertheless, deal decisively with even the most severe cases. As more sophistication has developed among legal authorities on child abuse and neglect, the careful use of appropriate legal proceedings to benefit the child and reduce unnecessary harm to the family and child has become more common. The health care professional can help legal authorities become aware of the need for a legal response attuned as much as possible to the child's needs.

Legal Responsibilities of the Health Care Professional

Frequent questions for any health care professional confronted with child abuse or neglect are: How do I know what abuse and neglect are from a legal perspective? Won't reporting or other involvement lead me into legal liability for errors, such as invasion of privacy? The definitional problem is addressed here first, because the discussion of how working definitions are developed and applied should alleviate concerns about legal liability in cases that are unclear or only suspected. Given this foundation, the ensuing discussion of potential legal liability demonstrates that the average, well-meaning, and reasonably trained health care professional has much more to fear from failing to respond to the child's situation than from becoming involved in a legally mandated and considered process of diagnosis and reporting. Later in this chapter the vulnerability of the health care professional involved either in failure to obtain consent or in inappropriate treatment where parental care is not a question is reviewed, followed by a discussion of the issues surrounding confidentiality.

Defining and "Proving" Child Abuse and Neglect

The statutory definitions of child abuse and neglect vary from state to state, but the differences are not great for the reporting professional's purposes. Briefly, this is so because the professional needs only to suspect child abuse, not prove it, and because the definitions depend practically on reasonable judgment that a particular child has been mistreated or neglected. For the nonprofessional these judgments are based on experience and a sense of fairness. For the professional there is the additional knowledge, acquired from training, of the causes and results of trauma and neglect. The definitions proposed in the Department of Health, Education and Welfare's draft Model Child Protection Act (DHEW, 1977) reflect to a great extent existing state laws:

(*a*) "Child" means a person under the age of 18.
(*b*) An "abused or neglected" child means a child whose physical or mental health or welfare is harmed or threatened with harm by the acts or omissions of his parent or other person responsible for his welfare.
(*c*) "Harm" to a child's health or welfare can occur when the parent or other person responsible for his welfare:

(*i*) inflicts or allows to be inflicted, upon the child, physical or mental injury, including injuries sustained as a result of excessive corporal punishment; or

(*ii*) commits or allows to be committed, against the child, a sexual offense, as defined by state law; or

(*iii*) fails to supply the child with adequate food, clothing, shelter, education (as defined by state law), or health care, though financially able to do so, or offered financial or other reasonable means to do so; for the purposes of this Act, "adequate health care" includes any medical or non-medical remedial health care permitted or authorized under state law; or

(*iv*) abandons the child as defined by state law; or

(*v*) fails to provide the child with adequate care, supervision or guardianship by specific acts or omissions of a similarly serious nature requiring intervention of the child protective service or a court.

(*d*) "Threatened harm" means a substantial risk of harm.

(*e*) "A person responsible for a child's welfare" includes the child's parent, guardian, foster parents, an employee of a public or private residential home, institution or agency; or the person legally responsible for the child's welfare in a residential setting.

(*f*) "Physical injury" means death, or permanent or temporary disfigurement or impairment of any bodily organ.

(*g*) "Mental injury" means an injury to the intellectual or psychological capacity of a child as evidenced by an observable, substantial impairment in his ability to function within his normal range of performance and behavior, with due regard to his culture.

The precise definition of child abuse and neglect varies from state to state, but this illustration is useful for showing that even the most developed definitions leave much unstated. These definitions, for example, do not say how much "harm" is too much. They do not explain what is "adequate" food, shelter, or health care. These terms are measured as a case is brought into the protective services or judicial systems. Community standards and professional knowledge determine how much harm is unacceptable. For example, when a child is killed, or has a leg fractured by rough handling, there is likely to be little question in the minds of professionals, judges, or ordinary citizens that harm has been done. If the injury is less understood by the public, as with a retinal bleed induced by shaking, nonorganic failure-to-thrive, or a frenum lacerated by forceable feeding, professional testimony will be needed to explain both the etiology and implications to the child of these types of harm.

A judge or jury ultimately decides, if the question is disputed, whether harm has been of a degree unacceptable by reasonable or perhaps even minimal community standards. The same approach ultimately "defines" what is adequate food, shelter, or medical and dental care, even though an occasional statute or case decision may be more specific. Thus, the statute may say that nonorganic failure-to-thrive is included within the meaning of child abuse and neglect. This still requires, however, that professionals be able to provide information about a child's condition, the etiology and consequences of the condition, the alternative interventions available and the probable consequences of each, and other information which will permit a determination of whether what has occurred presents unreasonable dental care of the child based on community standards.

Fortunately, for the dental professional faced with bruising, traumatized teeth, venereal lesions, or other signs of nonaccidental trauma or neglect, certainty is not required of the initial diagnosis. Only suspicion is required to make a report in all states and, in fact, mere suspicion of child abuse and neglect makes reporting mandatory. Lawyers, not the health care provider, must "prove" child abuse or neglect if it becomes necessary. Careful intervention by the health care provider with the help of social services and the court, if necessary, will often permit the child to be treated without the case ever having to be adjudicated. Such negotiated settlements often are possible.

Two more definitional examples might be helpful. Corporal punishment in the home is permitted in all 50 states as long as it is "ordinary" or "reasonable." Along a continuum of punishment, almost no communities would impose the label of "abuse" if a parent used an open hand and left no bruises on the buttocks of an adolescent. But using a belt on and bruising a four-year-old, not only on the buttocks but on the lower back, would make most judges and jurors want to know about the actual damage or potential damage to internal organs occurring from such actions. A parent who used the buckle end of the belt around the face of an infant, even if he/she felt justified, should not be surprised if every community considers such punishment unacceptable by local standards. The prospect of blindness, deafness, scarring and retardation, unless the facts proved otherwise, would greatly concern most citizens confronted with the final description of "punishment."

Dental neglect again involves questions of when the courts will order intervention based on understanding of law and professional findings. The court likely will order treatment if: a health condition is likely to lead to imminent death or serious impairment; there are few contradictions to the procedure; the prospects for full health are excellent, assuming intervention; the intervention has proven to have a high probability of success; it is an older child who agrees, or a very much younger child, for whom substitute judgment always must be made; *and* there is unanimity among professionals about the proposed procedure. If any of these factors is absent, the chance for ordered intervention is decreased but still possible. At least one court has sustained a neglect petition where a child had untreated fractured teeth and dental caries (*Mtr. of Gregory S.*, 1976).

"Dental neglect," with no further definition given, must be reported in Wisconsin and New York (Wis. Stat. Ann., 1979, New York Family Act, 1975). The strongest case for intervention, obviously, would be an odontogenic infection, oral cancer or other condition with a high probability of severe impairment or death of the child. Perhaps the most likely types of dental care neglect would be those involving nursing bottle caries; numerous, uncared-for caries or fractured teeth; or other significant dental problems. These must be accompanied by signs of severe, overall parental *neglect,* as opposed to a financial inability to provide care. From a practical perspective, the dental professional should not hesitate to report suspected neglect if he/she believes no reasonably prudent parent would fail to have the child treated under the circumstances presented.

The other logical possibility for neglect, is that the parent agrees to a treatment procedure that is unnecessary and harmful. Practically, human subject experimentation would seem the only likely instance of this type of neglect. Human experimentation is tightly regulated, however, especially when any federal funds are involved (DHEW, 1977).

Sources of Professional Liability

A medical or dental professional can be held liable for negligence or breach of law on several counts, including failure to diagnose child abuse and neglect, failure to report suspected child abuse and neglect, failure to obtain informed consent, failure to treat with acceptable methods, and breaches of confidentiality. It is important to remember that there are protections matching each of these potential sources of liability and that the reasonable professional who understands basic responsibilities and performs within ordinary limits of professional care can largely immunize his/her practice from malpractice recoveries in this area.

Failure to Diagnose

Medical and dental journals are publishing increasingly more articles on basic aspects of diagnosing and treating child abuse and neglect (Sherman, 1970; Laskin, 1973; Benusis, 1978; Beaver and McClendon, 1979; Malecz, 1979; Ellerstein, 1981). Some of these aspects warrant comment because they are associated with the clear risk of failure to diagnose. Because diagnosing child abuse and neglect can require more than physical findings (BEBR, 1980), the dental professional must be prepared to focus on history-taking and to seek consultations from specialists in dentistry and other disciplines. In addition to standard history-taking, it is essential to observe patient and parent behavior and to record statements tending to support or call into question possibilities of nonaccidental trauma, particularly the unadorned, first explanation of the circumstances of the injury or condition observed. Explanations that change and/or are inconsistent with the injuries or condition are, of course, classic findings in child abuse or neglect cases.

Consultations with multi-disciplinary child protection teams are becoming a standard medical practice (Schmitt, 1978) that dentists should not ignore. Failure to refer a case for diagnosis or treatment where a reasonably prudent professional would infer that the case may be beyond his/her immediate expertise, can create the basis for malpractice liability. One example of specialized knowledge is bitemark evidence, which has been developed largely by forensic odontologists, whose testimonies are now being accepted even in criminal proceedings in at least one state (Beckstead et al., 1979; *People v. Watson,* 1977; *People v. Sloan,* 1978; *People v. Gerschen,* 1977). Another example is medical examination, which can provide radiographic, developmental, or other visual signs or symptoms of abuse or neglect.

Failure to Report

Generally, the most open-and-shut liability case can be made for failure to report when a child is injured after being seen by a professional who diagnosed or should have diagnosed child abuse or neglect but failed to report it. All 50 states and several U.S. territories have enacted laws mandating the reporting of child abuse and neglect, with either civil or criminal penalties, or both, for failure to do so (ECS, 1979). Dentists specifically are mandated to report in Alaska, Alabama, Arkansas, Colorado, Illinois, Kansas, Maryland, Nebraska, Nevada, New York, North Dakota, South Dakota, Tennessee, Utah, Wyoming, West Virginia, the District of Columbia, Guam, and American Samoa. Medical personnel in general are required to report in 45 of the 50 states, and everyone, including professionals, must report in the remaining five states (Besharov, 1978).

In most instances of malpractice, the judge or jury must be convinced that there is a standard of professional care applicable and that the standard requires better performance than was achieved. If a law requires a certain performance, then the failure to perform that duty is automatically negligence, legally termed negligence per se. The attorney for a subsequently injured child must show that, but for the professional's act, the child would not have been hurt or reinjured. There is no need to show that the act of not reporting was negligence, only that the report was not made. In *Landeros v. Flood,* the 1976 case in which the California Supreme Court ruled that a physician can be negligent in failing to diagnose and report child abuse and neglect, a physician was relieved of liability by a jury only on the basis that he was not negligent in failing, on the facts of the case, to diagnose child abuse and neglect. There have been other, out-of-court, settlements, and criminal and civil prosecutions for failure to report are frequently noted in newspapers and professional journals (Besharov, 1978).

The fact that child abuse and neglect need only be "suspected" is an aid to the health care professional who wants to be safe in reporting. The health care professional who hesitates, in order to "protect" a family long-known and treated, however, is more at risk for liability if the child is injured. In assuming sole responsibility for trying to keep a child from being reinjured, the health care professional has to consider whether he/she wants to be in a position of having to show that child abuse or neglect was never suspected.

Fears about breaching confidentiality are understandable, but it can be shown that reporting of suspected child abuse and neglect does not fit within the usual framework of professional-client privilege of confidentiality. Concerns about the discomforts of dealing with parents are more realistic obstacles to reporting than is confidentiality.

Failure to Obtain Informed Consent

Liability arising from a failure to obtain informed consent raises the issue of the dental professional's abusive or neglectful actions toward the child patient rather than the parent's actions or omissions. Lack of informed consent has been a burgeoning area of medical malpractice law since the early 1970s (*Woods v. Brumlop,* 1962; *Canterbury v. Spence et al.,* 1972; *Cobbs v. Grant,* 1972; *Garone v. Robert's Technical and Trades School Inc.,* 1975). The safest standard to follow is providing the parent and the child, if he/she is reasonably competent, all of the information that a prudent patient in the same or similar circumstance would want before agreeing to or refusing a diagnostic or treatment procedure.

Alternative, lesser standards are to provide the parent and patient with what a reasonably prudent dental professional in the community or a reasonably prudent dental professional following national standards would. These latter standards reflect the view that health professionals can inform a patient what he/she judges is in the patient's interest, a view decreasingly accepted in the courts. Only if the parent/patient has knowingly waived the right to know what is involved can the professional not divulge risks, consequences, and alternatives to a procedure. Arguably, there cannot be a "knowing" waiver where a child is involved, hence the parent must know and consider what is involved to fulfill reasonable parental duties.

Treatment Malpractice and Wrongful Practices by the Dental Professional
Failure to exercise due care and treatment as a basis for malpractice recovery is encompassed by standard dental legal treatises (Howard and Parks, 1973; Miller, 1970; Sarner, 1963). Malpractice for failure to report as a part of necessary treatment for child abuse or neglect has already been discussed in this chapter. The child who is negligently handled by a treating health professional is in basically the same position as an adult. That is, he/she can sue for the negligent act of commission or omission that proximately harmed the patient. Children, however, are often given more time under statutes of limitations to sue for recovery. This is allowed on the principle that a limitation on recovery should not be held against an incompetent victim until the victim can reasonably be expected to discover the harm and/or negligence.

A special issue related to child abuse and neglect is the use of ancillary techniques of patient control, techniques that may no longer be acceptable to other health professionals and/or the public. The facts surrounding the incident(s) and community standards determine whether these practices constitute professional child abuse and neglect. Examples are corporal punishment, physical restraints, and restraint discipline techniques, such as the hand-over-mouth (HOM) technique.

"The physican or dentist has no special privilege to apply corporal punishment—spanking or slapping—to minor patients," writes S.L. Miller (1977). "There must be some expressed or implied consent. Any non-consensual, offensive touching is battery, unless it is justified, for example, by self-defense." Two cases illustrate the principles underlying Miller's statement. A pediatrician struck a four-year-old child severely on the thigh in order to make her lie still while he removed sutures from her toe. The bruises were still evident three weeks later. The trial court awarded $500 for assault and battery, which was reduced to $250 by the appellate court because there was no permanent damage. The physician's defense that he had acted pursuant to his professional judgment to maintain order was rejected (*Burton v. Leftwich,* 1960).

In the other case, a 23-month-old patient clamped her teeth on the finger of the physician's finger through to the bone, causing a spurt of blood as he was attempting to examine her lacerated tongue. After vainly shouting and trying to extract his finger using a tongue depressor, he slapped the child's cheek once. The District of Columbia court ruled that the act was rash, but not malicious, and that it was done in self-defense. The blow was not severe and the child was not injured. The court indicated that such cases should be decided on at least three characteristics of the force: necessity, amount, and the manner in which it was applied (*Mattocks v. Bell,* 1963).

Hand-over-mouth (HOM) techniques are arguable as assault and battery if used without consent and, when an adolescent is involved, it is doubtful the adolescent's wishes could be overridden by parental consent (Healy and Nowak, 1977). Physical restraints can raise claims of false imprisonment or assault and battery, with lack of consent raising another theory for recovery. Physical restraint would probably have to be justified, assuming full informed consent, as the only reasonable alternative available. Physical restraint might have been the best alternative in three cases where the patient's reaction to general anesthesia created special risks (ABA, 1981). These wrongful death cases were associated with anesthesia complications in dental practice.

Breach of Confidentiality

By statute (e.g., Ill. Ann. Stat., 1977; N.Y. Civ. Prac. Law, 1976) or case law, state laws impose a duty on all professionals not to divulge information about their patients or clients to others. In ordinary practice consultations among professionals occur. In these situations the professionals consulted are assumed not "part of the public." However, information unnecessary for a diagnosis, although difficult to prejudge, should not be shared even with another professional, especially if "publication" to those not involved in the case might occur and cause damage to the patient. An example of clear breach of confidentiality is unconsented release of identifying information to the news media, absent a court order.

Special Protections for Health Care Professionals

To encourage professionals to report suspected child abuse and neglect (Paulsen, 1967) legislators have created specific incentives and safeguards including (*a*) grants of immunity for mandated reporters in all 50 states (Besharov, 1978), (*b*) specific powers to obtain photographs and radiographs in 18 states, and (*c*) abrogation of privileged communications in 33 states by 1977 (ECS, 1977).

Reporting in Good Faith

There is consensus among lawyers knowledgeable in the area of child abuse and neglect that a person mandated to report where there is a reasonable basis for suspecting child abuse and neglect is not and would not be liable under ordinary case law, or "common law," for the action of reporting. Reporting possible harm to a child is considered a service normally contributing to the general well-being of society by the legislature requiring reporting. According to Foster and Freed (1966), "[T]he common law and all of our decisional authority already confers such immunity, and there is no American case that even suggests that there may be a liability for a good faith report of the kind required by battered child statutes" (Besharov, 1978; *see also* McCoid, 1965). The term "good faith" is a legal term for acting honestly or without malice. In other words, the reporting professional would not be protected if, *and only if,* he/she lied or was willfully and wantonly reckless with the truth.

Here immunity means that neither criminal nor civil complaints would be upheld if brought against the professional. For example, malpractice or defamation complaints could be filed against the reporter, but would be dismissed unless evidence of bad faith, i.e., deliberate lying or reckless disregard for the truth was also introduced. If a person who knew or should have known that a report was not malicious brings charges against the reporter, the reporter can sue for misuse of process on grounds that the person suing was bringing a vexacious law suit against the reporter in contradiction of public policy and equity.

Mandated reporters in most states are presumed to have acted in good faith, putting all the burden on the person unhappy with the report to prove it was both wrong and wrongful. As discussed above, it is not necessary for the reporter to prove child abuse and neglect, it is only necessary to show there was a reasonable basis to suspect child abuse and neglect at the time of reporting, which by necessity is early in the investigative process. Certainly, the ordinary professional has every possible safeguard and incentive to encourage reporting.

Health care professionals experienced in handling child abuse and neglect emphasize the need to report, based on the law. They stress that reporting should be accompanied by an explanation to parents of the professional's liability when he/she does not report "suspected" or "possible" child abuse and neglect. These professionals assure the family that they want to work with them and help them no matter what results from further evaluation, and that they will continue to be available to them (Schmitt, 1978a; Schmitt and Kempe, 1975; Helfer, 1974). They use the law to the advantage of children, families, and their own practices (see Chapter 9).

Consent for Examinations, Photographs, and Radiographs

It remains common practice for dental professionals to diagnose and treat patients relying on oral or implied consent, rather than obtaining full informed consent with written confirmation. This may change, for reasons discussed above, as the implications of medical malpractice decisions are better understood. Usual procedures require consent, and in the sense that one possible dental diagnosis is nonaccidental trauma and another is dental neglect, the consent to conduct an ordinary dental examination and provide dental treatment also should be sufficient to examine for signs of child abuse or neglect. Perhaps the most important caution would be to not proceed in the areas arguably belonging strictly to medical diagnosis, such as full body examination or full body radiographs. These can best be handled by medical consultation and will relieve the dental professional from having to establish medical credentials justifying nondental examination and diagnosis.

In general, consent should be sought when radiographs, photographs, or other additional documentation (e.g., study cast impressions) are deemed necessary for complete diagnostic or treatment records. A number of states have provided statutes waiving the need for parent or legal custodian consent for photographs and/or radiographs when they are necessary to document suspected child abuse or neglect (ECS, 1979).

Since photographs are not physically hazardous, their use for documentation can be argued to be a normal part of record-keeping requiring no special consent if carried out incidental to documentation of suspected, nonaccidental trauma. When consent to photography or radiography is reasonably approached as necessary for complete documentation, is then refused, and no express permission to photograph or radiograph is found in state statutes, the dental professional should be aware of two other possibilities. Some states permit seeking a court order for temporary custody of a child present before a health care professional who reasonably suspects child abuse or neglect. All states, however, permit seeking of orders for medical examinations of parties in a law suit. An alternative becomes available once a report is made and child protective services have begun investigating or have filed the petition alleging abuse or neglect. The exact procedure depends on state law, but the dental professional should indicate the need for more complete physical data collection than was possible, when he/she initially reports such cases.

Abrogation of Certain Duties of Confidentiality

As previously noted, professionals are normally not permitted to divulge information about clients absent without a release by the client or by someone with authority to authorize a release. In the area of child abuse and neglect, 33 states have enacted statutes specifically abrogating the privilege for mandated reporters or for all professional-client privileges.

Even when not safeguarded by a provision abrogating the confidentiality privilege, the law mandating reporting presumably overrides any prior privilege as it pertains to child abuse and neglect cases. Consideration of the usual practices of intradisciplinary and interdisciplinary consultations in questionable, difficult, or complex cases further suggests that reporting child abuse and neglect cases constitutes appropriate and prudent professional performance. Using multidisciplinary child protection teams to staff child abuse cases is, in fact, increasingly becoming the medical standard for performance. Clearly, consultation with legal authorities should be included as part of the interdisciplinary evaluation whenever there is any question about legal procedures.

The Dental Professional as Child Advocate

While mandated responsibilities are the minimal the dental professional must fulfill, more can and often must be done if children and families are to be helped. The dental professional needs to examine his/her role in caring for a child. The previous discussion on the dental professional's role in the legal process was included to help dental professionals become informed "consumers" of the law on behalf of children and families. The law can be a therapeutic tool, especially in addressing the social/medical/psychological problem of child abuse and neglect.

Patient Care

Hesitation to report suspected child abuse and neglect addressed by mandatory reporting laws seems to reflect confusion as to whom is being treated when child abuse or neglect is suspected. When a dental practitioner is working with a child, the child's needs must, of course, be a primary concern. Treatment of a patient endangered by the environment is superficial unless the environmental hazards are addressed. It does not help the child to avoid diagnosing or treating child abuse or neglect. By the same token, the family needing help cannot be reached until the problem is recognized fully. By understanding that a child may require advocacy as part of evaluation and treatment intervention, the dental practitioner takes a necessary step towards comprehensive patient care. Too often the question is: If not the health professional, who will advocate for the child?

Participation in the Legal Process

In addition to reporting and involvement with the child protection team, there are other aspects of the legal and protective process the dentist acting as advocate should know about. In 1978 Besharov reported central registries in 47 states and the District of Columbia. Utah has established a registry since then, leaving Minnesota and New Mexico the only states without them. Registries can be resources for statistics and/or help diagnosing and monitoring cases. They often make available to professionals treating a child any records of previously reported child abuse or neglect in the family.

One way of keeping the legal system accountable is for the dentist to be sure that a judge hears evidence of abuse and neglect. The decision to criminally prosecute, as noted above, rests with the district or state's attorney, but under some state statutes civil action may be initiated by any person having reason to believe a child is abused or neglected (e.g., Colo. Rev. Stat., 1973). Consultation with an attorney will help the dental practitioner know what avenues are available. Unfortunately, law and lawyers may represent obstacles to the child's protection. For example, an inexperienced lawyer may assert that no precedent exists for a certain type of legal action, that there is insufficient evidence to proceed, or that legal intervention will be damaging to the child, who may have to be a witness. A specialist in child abuse and neglect law will often provide different answers than those of a general practitioner. By asking questions, self-education about the law, and perseverence, the dental practitioner might cause the legal system to respond when, because of lack of money, lack of concern, or desire for political expediency, it is reluctant to.

Law as a Therapeutic Aid

A report of suspected child abuse and neglect risks mistakes of incompetence, overreaction, and any error that men and women are capable of making in the effort to do good. These are, of course, risks in almost every dental and medical procedure. Use of the appropriate alternative legal intervention, involvement of competent and well-intentioned professionals from a multidisciplinary perspective, and a focus on treatment needs of both parents and children will generally produce good results.

While legal intervention carries risks, it is apparent that in many cases no other means is available to assure child protection. A nonrandomized study reported that families court-ordered into treatment were five times more likely to successfully complete treatment than those for whom a voluntary arrangement was allowed (Wolfe et al., 1980). In each stage of child abuse and neglect case management, the law is important in assuring protection for children. Good practice by the dental profession requires participation in the societal effort to assure protection of all children.

References

American Bar Association (ABA): Amer. Bar Assoc. J. 67:1612, 1981.

Beaver, H.A. and McClendon, E.J.: The Dentist's Responsibility in Child Abuse and Neglect. J. Mich. Dent. Assoc. 97:133, 1979.

Becker, D.B.; Needleman, H.L.; and Kotelchuck, M.: Child Abuse and Dentistry: Orofacial Trauma and Its Recognition by Dentists. J. Am. Dent. Assoc. 97:24, 1978.

Beckstead, J.W.; Dawson, R.D.; Giles, W.S.: Review of Bite-Mark Evidence. J. Am. Dent. Assoc. 99:69, 1979.

Benusis, K.: Child Abuse: What the Dentist Should Know. Dent. Assist. 47:22, 1978.

Besharov, D.J.: The Legal Aspects of Reporting Known and Suspected Child Abuse and Neglect. Vill. L. Rev. 23:458, 1978.

Bureau of Economic and Behavioral Research (BEBR): Report on the Dentist's Responsibility in Recognizing and Reporting Child Abuse. Chicago: The Council on Dental Practice, Am. Dental Assoc., 1980.

Burton v. Leftwich, 123 So. 2d. 766 (La. App., 1960).

Canterbury v. Spence et al., 464 F. 2d. 772 (D.C. Cir., 1972).

Cobbs v. Grant, 104 Cal. Rptr. 505, 8 Cal. 3rd 229, 502 P. 2d 1 (1972).

Colorado Revised Statutes. 19-3-101 (2) (1973).

Davis, G.R.; Domoto, P.K.; and Levy, R.L.: The Dentist's Role in Child Abuse and Neglect. J. Dent. Child. 46:185, 1979.

Department of Health, Education, and Welfare (DHEW): Model Child Protection Act with Commentary. Draft, Aug. 1977.

Department of Health, Education, and Welfare (DHEW), National Commission for the Protection of Human Subjects of Biomedical and Behavioral Research: Report of Recommendations and Research Involving Children, DHEW Publ. No. (OS) 77-004, 1977.

Education Commission of the States (ECS): Trends in Child Abuse and Neglect Reporting Statutes. Denver: ECS, 1977.

Education Commission of the States (ECS): Trends in Reporting Laws. Denver: ECS, 1979.

Ellerstein, N.S.: Child Abuse and Neglect: A Medical Reference. New York: John Wiley & Sons Inc., 1981.

Finlay v. Finlay, 148 N.E. 624 (N.Y., 1925).

Fontana, V.J.: The Maltreated Child: The Maltreatment Syndrome in Children. Springfield, Ill.: Charles C. Thomas, 1964.

Foster, H.H. and Freed, D.J.: Battered Child Legislation and Professional Immunity. Am. Bar Assoc. J. 52:1071, 1966.

Garone v. Robert's Technical and Trades School Inc., 366 N.Y.S. 2d 129 (N.Y. Sup. Ct., 1975).

Gordon, J.E.: Control of Communicable Diseases in Man. New York: American Public Health Association, 1965.

Griswold v. Connecticut, 381 U.S. 479 (1965).

Healy, A. and Nowak, A.J.: Management of Children by Health Professionals. Iowa City: University of Iowa Press, 1977.

Helfer, R.E.: The Responsibility and Role of the Physician. In Helfer, R.E. and Kempe, E.H. (ed.) The Battered Child. (2nd ed.). Chicago: University of Chicago Press, 1974.

Howard, W.W. and Parks, A.L.: The Dentist and the Law. (3rd ed.). St. Louis: The C.V. Mosby Co., 1973.

Illinois Annotated Statutes, Ch. 51, § 5.1 (3) (Smith-Hurd Supp. 1977).

In re Gault, 387 U.S. 1 (1967).

Jacobson v. Massachusetts, 197 U.S. 11 (1905).

Landeros v. Flood, 131 Cal. Rptr. 69, 17 Cal. 3d 399, 551 P. 2d 389 (1976).

Laskin, D.M.: The Battered-Child Syndrome. Oral Surg. 31:93, 1973.

Malecz, R.E.: Child Abuse: Its Relationship to Pedodontics. A Survey. J. Dent. Child. 46:193, 1979.
Mattocks v. Bell, 194 A. 2d 307 (D.C. App., 1963).
McCoid, A.H.: The Battered Child and Other Assaults Upon the Family. Minn. L. Rev. 50:1, 1965.
Meyer v. Nebraska, 262 U.S. 390 (1923).
Miller, R.: Legal Issues Involved in Child Maltreatment. In Healy, A. and Novack, A.J. (ed.) Management of Children by Health Professionals. Iowa City: University of Iowa Press, 1977.
Miller, S.L.: Legal Aspects of Dentistry. New York: G.P. Putnam's Sons, 1970.
Matter of Gregory S., 85 Misc. 2nd 846, 38 N.Y.S. 2nd 620 (1976).
National Center on Child Abuse and Neglect (NCCAN): Study Findings: National Study of the Incidence and Severity of Child Abuse and Neglect. Washington, D.C.: U.S. Dep. Health and Human Services, Publ. No. (OHDS) 81-30325., 1981.
New York Civ. Prac. Law. §§ 4504, 4505, 4507, 4058 (McKinney Supp., 1976).
New York Family Act, § 1012 (f) (McKinney, 1975).
Paulsen, M.G.: Child Abuse Reporting Laws: The Shape of the Legislation, Colum. L. Rev. 67:1, 1967.
Paulsen, M.G.: The Legal Framework for Child Protection, Colum. L. Rev. 66:679, 1966.
Paulsen, M.G.: The Law and Abused Children. In Helfer, R.E. and Kempe, C.H. (ed.) The Battered Child. (2nd ed.). Chicago: University of Chicago Press, 1974, p. 174.
People v. Gerschen, Stanislau County California, pretrial Nov. 1977.
People v. Slone, 143 Cal. Rptr. 61, 76 Cal. App. 3rd 611 (1978).
People v. Watson, 142 Cal. Rptr. 134, 75 Cal. App. 3rd 384 (1977).
Pierce v. Society of Sisters, 268 U.S. 510 (1925).
Prince v. Massachusetts, 321 U.S. 158 (1944).
Robertson, P.: Home as a Nest: Middle-Class Childhood in 19th Century Europe. In deMause, L. (ed.) The History of Childhood. New York: The Psycho History Press, 1974.
Sarner, H.: Dental Jurisprudence. Tampa: W.F. Poe Assoc., 1963.
Schmitt, B.D. Battered Child Syndrome (Child Abuse and Neglect). In Kempe, C.H., et al. (ed.) Current Pediatric Diagnosis and Treatment. Los Altos: Lange Medical Publishers, 1978a.
Schmitt, B.D. (ed.): The Child Protection Team Handbook: A Multidisciplinary Approach to Managing Child Abuse and Neglect. New York: Garland, 1978b.
Schmitt, B.D. and Kempe, C.H.: Child Abuse: Management and Prevention of the Battered Child Syndrome. Folia Traumatologica. Geigy, Basle, 1975.
Sherman, G.: The Abused Child—New York State. J. New York Dent. Assoc. 36:109, 1970.
Tarasoff v. Regents of the University of California, 17 Cal. 3rd 425, 551 P. 2d 334 (1976).
Wisconsin Statutes Annotated, 48.981 (1) (d) (West, 1979).
Wolfe, D.A.; Aragona, J.; Kaufman, K.; and Sandler, J.: The Importance of Adjudication in the Treatment of Child Abusers: Some Preliminary Findings. Child Abuse and Neglect 4:127, 1980.
Woods v. Brunlop, 71 N.M. 221, 337 P. 2d 520 (1962).

Chapter 12

Expert Testimony by Dentists in Child Abuse Litigation

Norman D. Sperber

Introduction

Litigation refers to a contest in a court of justice for the purpose of enforcing a right, whether it be a civil right or the right of society to be free of crime. Expert testimony is that of an expert witness: one whose training, skills, or knowledge are beyond that of the normal person, giving him/her privileges beyond those of an ordinary, or fact, witness.

The ordinary witness can testify to facts from his/her firsthand knowledge. For example, he/she can testify that he saw the blue car strike the green car in an automobile accident. The expert witness also testifies to facts he/she has observed. In addition, he/she is qualified to give an opinion before the trier of fact (judge or jury). The expert witness is not an advocate for either side, although he/she can be an advocate for his/her opinion. The attorneys who call in the experts are the advocates; the experts must remain independent and objective. The only responsibility of the expert witness is to aid the trier of fact in the search for the truth. Dentists and physicians by nature of their training are automatically expert witnesses within their professions, provided they maintain a current knowledge of their field.

The general dentist and the dental specialist may be confronted with nonaccidental injuries or unusual lesions in a pediatric patient and by legislative mandate become involved in reporting child abuse and testifying about observable injuries or lesions. The forensic dentist might also be called upon by various authorities to give expert testimony on nonaccidental or pattern injuries and/or unusual lesions. Mindful of the responsibilities as health professionals, this chapter will guide the dentist preparing to serve as an expert witness.

Qualifying the Expert Witness

After a dentist subpoenaed to give expert testimony in court has sworn to tell the truth, he/she will be asked questions designed to qualify him/her in the eyes of the judge. These can include name, business address, profession, education, speciality area, length of professional status and experience, professional memberships, publications, and previous testimony.

Procedure

The expert witness is first examined by the attorney who sought his services. Even the most inexperienced witness should have no apprehension at this point. He/She relates the facts and often opinions provided they are based on experience and training. Cross-examination may follow by the opposing attorney. Regardless of common belief, this need not be an ordeal if the expert simply realizes that the attorney is attempting to represent his client, not necessarily to ridicule the expert. Few attorneys are not courteous and appreciative of the expert's knowledge. The attorney who has called the dentist normally will prepare him/her for direct examination as well as redirect the questioning following cross-examination by opposing counsel.

Demeanor

The expert witness should listen carefully to each question and not attempt to analyze the attorney's strategy. Replies should be coherent and audible for recording by the courtroom reporter. Nonverbal communication is neither suitable nor acceptable in court, since all testimony must be carefully recorded by the court reporter.

It is important to avoid professional jargon unless it is certain the technical terms are well-understood by the jury and/or the officers of the court. "Lower jaw" should replace "mandible." The phrase "lower jaw, or mandible—as we call it" might also be used.

On the other hand, the dentist must never "talk down" to the trial participants or think the proceedings beneath his/her dignity because he/she is the authority on the subject. Indeed, it is because the dentist is the authority that he/she is mandated to educate the court. The expert must be patient when a question is asked repeatedly or when the answer seems obvious.

The dentist is not expected to give information not called for in a question. If he/she cannot answer the question as asked he should say so and state why. He should at all times be courteous to his questioners and address the judge as "Your Honor."

Testimony Concerning Evidence Collected by Others

Often the dentist will be called on to testify regarding evidence gathered by others. For example, a forensic dentist might in a homicide trial where the photographs and impressions of bite mark(s) were taken by law enforcement agents and the impressions of the suspect(s) dentition by other dentists. The demeanor of the dentist as an expert witness remains the same whether or not he/she personally collected the evidence.

Discharge of Duties

After the expert has testified and answered questions from both sides, and after all testimony has been heard, the "trier of fact"—the judge or jury—will consider the arguments of both sides to reach a verdict. The demands of society will have been met and the duties of the expert witness will be discharged.

Summary

The dentist preparing to testify as an expert witness should maintain the following professional perspective:

- The dentist is an expert witness.
- He/She must be objective and impartial.
- He/She must be dignified and cooperative.

Reference

Woolridge, E.D.: Legal Aspects of Forensic Medicine and Dentistry. Dent. Clin. North Am. 21:19, 1977.

Chapter 13

Violence in Adult Family Members

Kristin F. Robbins

Introduction

As an outgrowth of increased public awareness of child abuse, the more encompassing problem of family violence has been recognized. Professionals in many disciplines now provide a wide range of services to victims of family violence. The impact of family violence within our society must be reviewed in order for the dental professional to be effective in providing treatment made necessary by violence among family members.

The literature does little to elucidate the impact of family-related abuse on the dental practitioner. However, statistics from an initial study of physically abused women indicated that 20 percent of all reported physical injuries were to the face and head and had potentially serious dental consequences (Thoeunes, 1981). Many of these injuries are being treated by the dental practitioner.

This chapter tells how to appropriately manage patients of suspected or confirmed family violence. Nature, types, characteristics, and extent of family violence will be discussed, with emphasis on the diagnosis and treatment of adults with abuse-related injuries. Suggestions are made for physical assessment of injuries, appropriate treatment planning considerations, office management of abused patients, legal responsibility to report adult abuse-related injuries, and sources of support that can offer a wide range of services to both battered men and women.

Nature of Family Violence

The stereotype of the family is characterized by love, affection, emotional support, and gentleness. Yet anyone who has lived in a family structure has experienced conflicts and everyday stresses among family members. Families vary significantly in their abilities and skills to cope with and resolve these inevitable conflicts. Unfortunately for many, society generally believes that personal and family problems should be resolved only in the privacy of the home. As relationships suffer and stress, frustrations, and tensions increase, families often attempt to end conflicts with physical force.

Types

Violence occurring among family members can take a variety of expressions, the primary being physical and/or emotional. Physical violence can be kicking, hitting, shoving, slapping, choking, throwing objects, or using a weapon. Emotional abuse includes threatening violence, demeaning a family member, withholding affection, and extremely and irrationally criticizing. Emotional abuse can be more damaging than physical abuse to the victim.

Characteristics

Family violence can include abuse of children, partners, siblings, the elderly, and of parents by children. Several types of violence commonly occur simultaneously in an abusive family. Family violence usually is an intensely emotion-laden event that can be expected to recur and escalate in the future (Barnett et al., 1980).

Financial status is not a predictable indicator of violent behavior since its incidence varies only slightly between white- and blue-collar families. Family violence occurs in all socioeconomic, ethnic, racial, and age groups (Barnett et al., 1980). The problem is perhaps more visible in low-income families because lower-income groups more often seek treatment through public health agencies or other institutions well-informed about identification. Families that can afford to are more likely to seek abuse-related health care from the private sector, often because it is the traditional approach, is highly confidential, and requires the divulging of very little information. Social status is thus preserved and maintained. Not admitting that a problem exists makes not facing the problem much easier.

Extent

Cases of physical abuse in families are estimated at one to eight million per year (Strauss, 1978). In many American cities family-related disputes, disturbances, and homicides comprise a large percentage of all police-responded episodes.

Divorce is one of the remedies for those who choose not to tolerate spouse abuse. Not surprisingly, divorce litigation often verifies the extent of physical abuse. In many cases repeated physical abuse is listed as a complaint. Since family violence often occurs within the privacy of the home, statistically accurate documentation of physical abuse will always contain limitations.

Diagnosis of Family Violence in Dental Practice

The most common injuries from family violence include bruises; loosened, fractured, or missing teeth; and fractured bones. Physical assessment of all trauma patients should begin when they enter the dental office. The receptionist should be alert to behavior that might pertain to the cause of the trauma and should convey initial impressions to the dentist at once. Dental auxiliaries also should help to elicit maximum information about a suspicious case. It is recommended that a female assistant seat a female patient alone. An abusive adult accompanying his/her abused partner to the initial appointment might appear agitated, concerned, and nervous, and insist on being in the operatory during treatment. The accompanying person should remain in the reception area, however.

Battered women and elderly adults generally view themselves as helpless, often lying to dental personnel about the cause of the trauma. To minimize this, the female dental auxiliary can collect routine health data while establishing patient rapport. Direct, confidential questions regarding the cause of injury should be asked and the questioner's motives explained. This will allow the patient to communicate honestly with the dental auxiliary before having the opportunity to fabricate a story. The dentist, if male, should enter and repeat the questioning in a routine manner. If the dentist is female, the dental auxiliary need not ask any questions. If the patient is male, however, the dental auxiliary and dentist, regardless of gender, both should ask pertinent questions.

When a patient affirms physical abuse, the dental staff needs to be organized, calm, and prepared to respond to a potential crisis situation. The dental staff should have established a mechanism for obtaining assistance since it is not recommended that they deal directly with the abusing person concerning the crisis. Instead, their efforts should focus on managing the injuries of the victim. Dental office personnel should not give information in the presence of the suspected abuser, but should have the patient call back later when it is safe to do so. They can also be referred to other formal agencies for assistance.

Oral facial injuries in abused adults may be accompanied by other facial trauma or previous injuries. To evaluate for previous injuries, possible fractures, or other physical characteristics consistent with a history of trauma, it is recommended that, as a minimum, a complete periapical and panoramic radiographic survey be taken as early as possible. Although an emergency situation, a thorough intraoral and extraoral facial should be performed, checking carefully for inconsistencies in clinical findings and elicited history.

Considerations in Treatment Planning

After thorough physical assessment and diagnosis a treatment plan must be prepared. Incidents of abuse usually are not isolated, but are repeated regularly. While emergency treatment protocol is identical regardless of whether the trauma is accidental, restorative treatment planning in cases of abuse should be influenced by the repetitious nature of abuse. If possible, fixed prosthodontic procedures should be delayed until the person is no longer subject to possible injury. Removable prosthodontic therapy is preferred for the interim. Referral dentists giving treatment must be informed of the abuse situation so that appropriate decisions can be made during all phases of treatment.

Office Management and Reporting

While neither the health practices acts nor the criminal codes of most states require the dentist to report incidents of physical abuse in adults, it is a professional obligation to report abuse of adults under a similar protocol as outlined in a state's child protection laws. Local reporting protocols can be obtained from county social service agencies or health departments.

In some cases the abused person may require protection from the abuser. Their charts should be clearly marked, stipulating that no information, including that of the chart's existence, be given to anyone except the patient. Appropriate marks can be put on the payment ledger card each time the patient is treated for another trauma. Since an entire family is often included on one payment ledger card, this is an easy and confidential way to audit a family for violence. A family with several incidents of suspicious trauma should be carefully and systematically assessed for physical abuse in other members.

Progress notes in the dental chart should include probable date of the trauma, date of the office visit, specific nature of the injuries, responses to the questions on abuse, the radiographic survey, treatment rendered, referrals suggested, and drugs prescribed.

Tragically, abused women and elderly adults have little economic control in their lives and are often denied access to any sources of money. Therefore, payment arrangements should be finalized when the partner is present. Full payment at the time of service is recommended since when any guilt that might have prompted the office visit diminishes, the desire to pay the dental fee might be reduced as well.

Summary

The impact of family violence on the practice of dentistry is significant. Incidence of physical abuse injuries to the oral facial complex requires further research efforts. Diagnosing and treating victims of family violence should be approached using current theories on office management and reporting.

References

Barnett, E.R.; Pittman, C.B.; Ragan, C.K.; and Salus, M.K.: Family Violence: Intervention Strategies. U.S. Dep. of Health and Human Services Pub. No. (OHDS) 80-30258, Washington, D.C., 1980.

Strauss, M.A.: National Survey of Domestic Violence: Some Preliminary Findings and Implications for Future Research. Prepared for Hearings on Research into Domestic Violence, U.S. House of Representatives Subcommittee on Domestic and International Scientific Planning, Analysis and Cooperation, Feb. 14, 1978.

Thoeunes, N.: The Consequences of Geographic Mobility: The Social Networks of Battered Women. Ph.D. Thesis. Denver: Colorado Women's College Press, 1981.

Selected References

Gaylord, J.J.: Battered Wives. Med. Sci. Law 15:237, 1975.

Justice, B. and Justice, R.: The Abusing Family. New York: Human Sciences Press, 1976.

Viano, E. (ed.): Special Issue of Spouse Abuse and Domestic Violence. Victimology: An International Journal 2:416, 1978.

Walker, L.: The Battered Woman. New York: Harper and Row, 1979.

Chapter 14

Dental Neglect in Children

Peter K. Domoto

Introduction

Dental neglect is a global problem caused by a high prevalence of dental pathology coupled with an inaccessibility to dental health care. The lack of access to dental services can be caused by a broad spectrum of barriers. Some of the barriers are:

- Patient isolation
- Lack of financing for dental care
- Patient ignorance
- Lack of perceived value of oral health

This chapter will discuss the problem of dental neglect in children within the context of the above barriers and will suggest guidelines for identification and management of neglect cases.

The problem of dental neglect must be addressed within its layers of context. Hally et al.'s instructive model of child neglect (1980) can be modified to describe the specific complexities of dental neglect in children. The model can be paraphrased as follows:

The dentally neglected child is a member of a family residing in a particular neighborhood. Neighborhoods coalesce to form a community, which is part of a larger society. The society possesses economic and political variations, which it shares with its several communities. These economic and political variables, along with cultural values, including those of child rearing, largely determine the standards for dental care in a community. Family child-rearing practices, and economic and political factors in a society will affect both the identification and the reporting of dental neglect.

Definition

Dental neglect should be seen as part of the larger area of child neglect.

Child neglect occurs when a caretaker either deliberately or by extraordinary inattentiveness permits the child to experience present suffering and/or fails to provide the child with the essentials for developing his or her physical, intellectual, and emotional capacities.

Dental neglect in children can be defined as negligence or maltreatment that harms their oral health. Most often, dental neglect is an act of omission.

Indicators

Identifying dental neglect is more complex than identifying dental abuse. Bases for seeking and providing dental care vary widely throughout the world, making it difficult to develop a consensus regarding guidelines for identifying of dental neglect. The literature until now has been largely devoid of clear guidelines for such identification. The following indicators of dental neglect were, however, noted by Davis et al. in 1979:

- Untreated rampant caries easily detected by a lay person
- Untreated pain, infection, bleeding, or trauma affecting the oral facial region
- History of a lack of continuity of care in the presence of identified dental pathology

An accurate and sensitive history is essential to confirm the suspicion of child dental neglect. A key factor in determining dental neglect is the failure of the parent or guardian to obtain appropriate dental care for their child following identification of serious dental pathology. A multitude of omissions can and should be forgiven when, due to the aforementioned barriers, people are unaware of the processes and outcomes of oral disease. However, when pathosis has been clearly identified, treatment precisely explained, and significant barriers to care removed, failure to follow through on the prescribed treatment is dental neglect. This concept is consistent with accepted definitions of child neglect and reflects current standards in identifying medical care neglect (USDHEW, 1975; Frentz, 1975–1976; Davis et al., 1979; Clarke, 1980; Hally et al., 1980).

Impact of Neglect Statutes on Dental Practice

In states where medical and dental neglect are defined synonymously, there can be a significant and direct impact on dental practice. In these states, parents and caretakers are expected to seek prompt medical and dental care and are generally expected to observe appropriate disease prevention practices (Washington State, 1976). Parents are considered neglectful of the medical and dental needs of their children in the following instances (Davis et al., 1979):

- Failure to respond to notification of child's medical and dental needs with arrangements for care
- Response to notification of child's medical and dental needs with inappropriate care
- Failure to arrange for medical and dental supervision of a child who is noticeably injured or ill
- Failure to arrange for medical and dental supervision of a child suffering from a disease, disabling condition or injury when specific evidence of such is present

- Inappropriate utilization of health resources, e.g., preventing continuous or follow-up care by frequent changing of doctors, hospitals, or clinics

Negligence in the provision of dental care to children is a new concept emerging from child abuse legislation. Many issues must be addressed prior to establishing a dental neglect policy in a state. First, law enforcement agencies must respond to cases of dental neglect in a supportive manner. Second, child protection workers must have a range of resources in order to meet the neglected child's needs. Third, public and/or private community service agencies are needed to support the dentally neglected child. In this era of constrained and shrinking resources for social services, it is essential that public and private funds be channeled to serve real human needs. These funds should help make dental services accessible by financing dental care for the needy. Fourth, the dentist must be able to identify and manage cases of dental neglect. These issues also emphasize the need for an effective support system in the management of the dentally neglected child.

A Case History

The procedures one general practitioner used to provide emergency treatment to a 15-year-old female illustrates effective management of dental neglect (Davis et al., 1979). During the initial appointment, a permanent tooth was extracted because decay had progressed beyond the bifurcation of the root and was judged nonrestorable. A later, follow-up examination revealed no evidence of prior restorative therapy and the presence of rampant caries and excessive plaque accumulations. A large scar was also noticed on her neck. Upon inquiry the dentist was told this was due to drainage from abscessed teeth and had been open for many months before healing occurred. He discovered the mother had not sought treatment for the serious problem even though she was urged to by other members of her family.

An older married sister brought the patient for initial visits and obtained legal permission from the mother for treatment of the 15-year-old, a 17-year-old sister, and a 14-year-old brother. All three had rampant caries and wanted dental care. However, they had to travel a long distance to receive treatment, and transportation could not always be provided by the married sister. After efforts to contact the mother failed, the general dentist called the local child protective services, which provided transportation and other family support over a two-year period in which all three children received complete dental treatment.

Under state of Washington law, the dentist was required to report the suspected dental and nutritional neglect; and child protective services were legally bound to investigate and provide supportive services to the children and family in order to resolve the problem. This case shows that many kinds of support must be available for a beneficial outcome.

Recommendations for Policy Formulation

It is incumbent upon dentists to provide leadership in their respective states toward the formulation of dental neglect policy. Although scientific data is lacking, ample knowledge based on clinical experience, understanding of values, and common sense exists to provide a consensus for state and community policies on child dental neglect identification and management.

Recent publications in the medical/legal literature document the formulation of child neglect policy as related to medical care (Frentz, 1976; Goldstein et al., 1979; Clarke, 1980). Analysis of case law dealing with nonemergency treatment reveals a pattern of discretionary decisions, each weighing certain factors (Frentz, 1976). These are:

- The probable effect on the child's social, physical, and emotional well-being if treatment is allowed or denied
- The seriousness of the condition, the medical risks involved, and the probabilities of success as judged by competent medical opinion
- The reasonableness of parents' objections
- The wishes and cooperation of the child

Dental policy makers would be wise to incorporate these into their policies.

Neglect Statutes Invoked for Health Care

Health professionals must temper their enthusiasm to treat children when death is not an issue (Goldstein et al., 1979). Neglect statutes can be invoked in the name of health care to perform treatment procedures specified by health authorities yet not wanted by parent or child. Such inappropriate use of neglect laws violates family privacy and undermines parental autonomy (Goldstein et al., 1979). In recognition of the rights of both parent and child, the utmost care must be taken by the dentist to create a supportive context in which dental care can proceed. A sensitive and careful history-taking process is essential to initiate supportive dental services. Diagnostic findings and treatment plans should be clearly and precisely delineated in a nonjudgmental manner. Management of the care should be conducted in the least intrusive and most supportive way possible (Goldstein et al., 1979).

Summary

Untreated oral disease in children is a significant world health problem. It is unacceptable and frustrating to acknowledge the apparent state of dental neglect experienced by many children. With the preventive and therapeutic technology available today there should be effective dental disease control measures accessible to every child. Dentists, legislators, courts, and parents would do well to be guided by a primary and overriding concern for the well-being of children in formulating a policy of dental neglect identification and management.

References

Clarke, A.M.: The Choice to Refuse or Withold Medical Treatment. Creighton L. Rev. 13:795, 1980.

Davis, G.R.; Domoto, P.K.; and Levy, R.L.: The Dentist's Role in Child Abuse and Neglect. J. Dent. Child. 46:185–192, 1979.

Frentz, T.W.: Minors' Rights to Medical Care. J. Family L. 14:581, 1975–1976.

Goldstein, J.; Freud, A.; and Solnit, A.J.: Before the Best Interests of the Child. New York: The Free Press, 1979.

Hally, C.; Polansky, N.F.; and Polansky, N.A.: Child Neglect: Mobilizing Services. U.S. Dep. of Health and Human Services Pub. No. (OHDS) 80-30257, 1980.

U.S. Dep. of Health, Education and Welfare: Child Abuse and Neglect: The Problem and Its Management, Vol. 1, An Overview of the Problem. DHEW Pub. No. (OHD) 75-30073, Washington, D.C., 1975.

Washington State Dept. of Social and Health Services: Child Protective Services Manual H, Rev. 35. Seattle: DSHS, 1976.

Chapter 15

Cultural Health Practices Suspected as Child Abuse

Robert E. Primosch

Introduction

Recent published reports reveal the distress to parents falsely accused of child abuse. In London, a Nigerian mother was arrested on charges of child abuse after cutting the faces of her children with a razor blade and rubbing charcoal into the lacerations (Korbin, 1977). She was released after it was determined that she was attempting to assert tribal identity upon her children by practicing scarification, a tradition among the Yoruba tribe of rural Nigeria. In Vietnam, a father committed suicide in jail after being arrested for child abuse (Ahn, 1976). Evidently, the father had performed the folk medicine practice of Cao Gio, causing the hospitalization and death by pneumonia of his son.

Practically every culture has accepted methods of child rearing that can culminate in physical injury to the child. Since these may be misinterpreted as child abuse, additional guidelines would be useful to the health professional who is obligated legally and professionally to report all suspected cases of nonaccidental trauma. Currently, there is consensus that any well-accepted cultural practice that inflicts trauma without malice but out of true concern for the child's well-being does not constitute child abuse and should not be managed as such (Keller and Apthorp, 1977; Taylor and Newberger, 1979). This chapter will identify several cultural health practices that might be misinterpreted as child abuse and will discuss considerations for an international definition of child abuse.

Folk Remedies

Cultural health practices that have been suspected as child abuse usually have been the results of treatment by folk medicine. Folk remedies are established in tradition and generally found in underdeveloped societies of rural, agrarian background. Acceptance of folk remedies allows the practitioner to deal with the difficulties often encountered at the interface of two diverse cultures. The wide variations in cultures, along with the increased, worldwide mobility of populations, enhance the likelihood of cultural conflict and subsequent cases of mistaken suspicions of child abuse.

Folk medical systems are found throughout the United States in isolated sub-

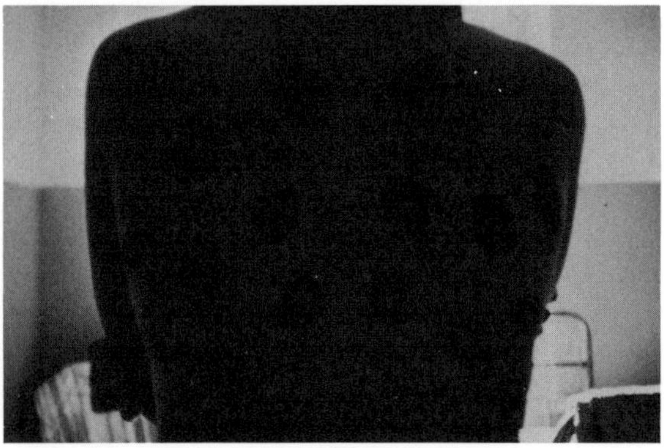

Fig. 15-1 Typical marks created by dry cupping. (Courtesy of Dr. Stephen K. Young)

cultures such as the Pennsylvania Dutch, Amish, Appalachian whites, Southern blacks, Louisiana Cajuns, Kansas farmers, New York City Puerto Ricans, and Californian Mexican-Americans. Among rural Southern blacks of low socioeconomic status, folk medicine beliefs are based on a mixture of African folklore, fundamentalist Christianity, and West Indian voodoo (Snow, 1974). These beliefs are based on attitudes that view the world as hostile, dangerous, and controlled by a punitive God. In turn, these attitudes breed distrust and create reliance on self-treatment.

Dry Cupping

One such method of self-treatment is the folk medicine practice of dry cupping, an ancient medical practice similar to acupuncture. Dry cupping, reported among Soviet and Mexican immigrants to the United States (Sandler and Haynes, 1978; Stoeckle and Carter, 1980), is a therapeutic technique for aches, pains, and congestion. Its effectiveness is believed to be the influence of a faith-based placebo. Dry cupping is inverting a cup or glass in which a small amount of alcohol has been ignited onto the unbroken skin overlying the affected part of the body. Suction occurs when the hot air in the cup cools, and leads to localized congestion of the skin that disappears within 2 to 3 days (Fig. 15-1). The purpose is to draw bad blood to the surface to relieve the congestion within. This practice differs from wet cupping where prior piercing of the skin leads to blood letting and scarification. Dry cupping is harmless and painless, unless wrongly applied. Burns rarely result. However, a case was reported where gasoline was substituted for alcohol and severe burns resulted from accidental spilling (Stoeckle and Carter, 1980).

Mollera Caida

A folk medicine belief called Mollera Caida, or fallen fontanel, is practiced by some Mexican-Americans (Guarnaschelli, 1972). Practitioners of Mollera Caida feel that illness is due to imbalances and disharmony among the four humors or when body parts move from their normal positions. Fallen fontanel or the downward displacement of the anterior fontanel may be caused by a fall or rapid removal of the nursing bottle from the mouth. The fallen fontanel creates a downward projection of the hard palate called "bolita," or little ball, and is believed to result in feeding problems, vomiting, diarrhea, and lethargy. Treatment for fallen fontanel consists of a series of four separate maneuvers that are essentially harmless. However, a two-month-old infant treated for fallen fontanel was reported to have developed a subdural hematoma caused by the abusive use of the fourth in the series of treatments (Guarnaschelli et al., 1972). This step ends with holding the infant upside down by the ankles with the crown of the head submerged in boiling water. While inverted, the infant is shaken vigorously and slapped on the soles of the feet.

Other Mexican-American Folk Remedies

Other Mexican-American folk practices include Mal Ojo, or evil eye; Susto, or magical fright; and Empacho, or surfeit (Sandler and Chan, 1978). Empacho is intestinal blockage believed to be caused by a bolus of food adhering to the stomach. The treatment often is not harmful and consists of a back massage and oral administration of castor oil. However, two case reports are available where infants were given metallic mercury orally by a "curadera," or Mexican folk doctor, for treatment of gastroenteritis (Geffner and Sandler, 1980). The oral mercury was aimed at dislodging the obstruction. Fortunately minimal toxicity occurred because metallic mercury is rarely absorbed.

Cao Gio

Cao Gio is a unique folk medicine practice popular among the people of rural Vietnam. Numerous recent reports are available describing the practice and its manifestations (Ahn, 1976; Gellis et al., 1976; Yeatman et al., 1976; Keller and Blair, 1976; Du, 1980; Primosch and Young, 1980). Recent awareness of this practice among American health care professionals and its ability to mimic child abuse was treated in a 1980 issue of *Time* magazine (Time Inc., 1980).

Cao Gio, which literally means "scratch the wind," is the abrasive rubbing of a coin across the oiled skin until ecchymoses appear. The practice is a routine first aid attempt to free the body of "bad winds" believed responsible for various physical ailments, including fever, headache, and convulsions, and is applied to the symptomatic area. The back, head, neck, and chest are common sites of application. At times a cloth might be substituted for a coin, or water will be used instead of aromatic ointments as a lubricating medium.

The trauma resulting from excessive rubbing can mimic child abuse, but it is painless and no complications are known to result. The orderly, bilateral, and linear patterns of the ecchymoses along with taking an adequate history help distinguish this practice from child abuse (Figs. 15-2 and 15-3). A good Cao Gio treatment should leave only a temporary redness to the skin without ecchymosis formation.

A recent survey of 50 Vietnamese immigrants indicated that this practice was widely used and relieved symptoms (Yeatman, 1980). The attempt to stimulate

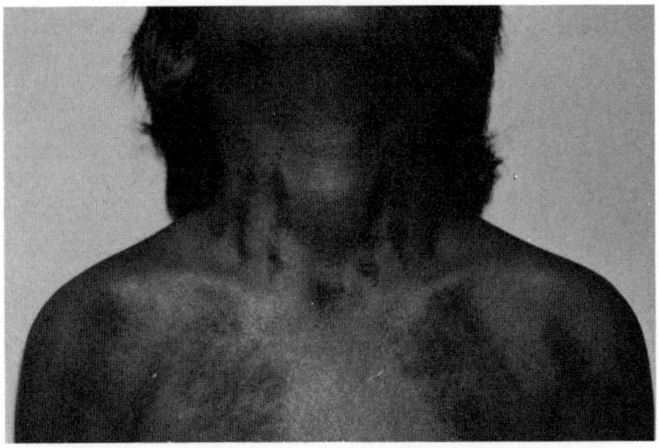

Figs. 15-2 and 15-3 The orderly, bilateral, and linear patterns of the ecchymoses created by Cao Gio mimic some lesions found in child abuse.

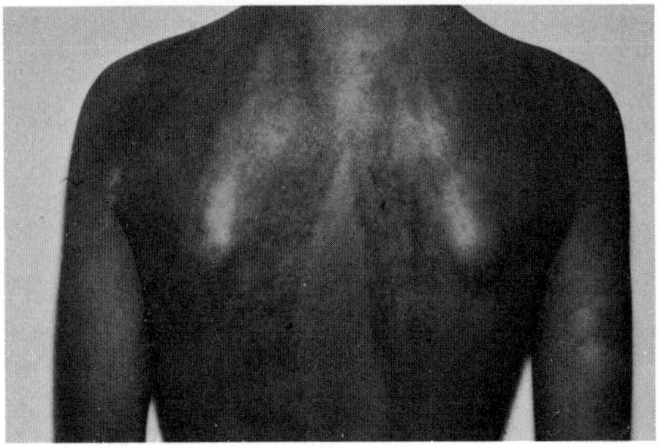

Figure 15-3

certain trigger points is considered a method of needless acupuncture. Stimulating nerve endings at certain points with pressure has similarities to the Chinese acupuncture meridians (Ho-Quang-Phuoc, 1981). It is believed that the Vietnamese adopted the principles from the Chinese and adapted the practice as a form of home self-treatment. Bat Gio, the pinching of certain points on the temples, forehead, and neck, is also adapted by the Vietnamese from Chinese acupuncture (Ho-Quang-Phuoc, 1981) (Fig. 15-4).

Cao Gio and Bat Gio are not child abuse and should not be managed as such. Because the lesions mimic child abuse but are not intended to do harm, the term ''pseudobattering'' is the best known label. Cao Gio should be discussed with the user in neutral terms to improve acceptance of and compliance with modern medical practices when truly needed.

Folk Remedies and Modern Health Care

Practitioners should be aware that patients' behavior may be adversely affected by their commitment to their belief system. Deeply ingrained folk beliefs about how to attain and maintain health will influence the doctor/patient relationship and

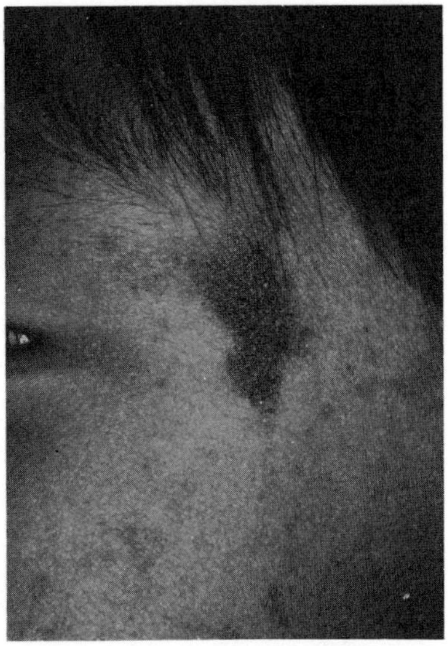

Fig. 15-4 The mark resulting from pinching the skin over the temples of this Vietnamese child was created during Bat Gio.

especially the degree to which the patient follows the doctor's orders. Superstitious beliefs can play a major role in health care delivery. By the time such individuals arrive for traditional medical treatment, it is probably as a last resort after every home remedy has been tried. Severe or last-resort home remedies can include the oral administration of kerosene, turpentine, moth balls, and carbon tetrachloride (Hughes, 1963; Snow, 1974). The dentist might observe direct manifestations of these.

Folk customs perceived necessary for group survival can become strongly incorporated into the culture. The Bedouin tribe in South Sinai, Israel, sanctions the removal of a child's uvula with a hot knife during the first year of life. The uvula is removed because it is believed that its absence will decrease thirst, a particularly acute problem in an area with a shortage of drinking water (Rubenstein, 1979). Because customs develop over time, people relinquish them only reluctantly. Accepted value systems of a culture become deeply ingrained, and disadvantaged people adhere particularly strongly to them. A cultural practice will disappear only when it becomes dysfunctional and no longer contributes to survival of the society.

Management of Folk Practices

Practitioners must be sensitive to the belief systems of their patients. When a folk medicine practice is encountered, the practitioner should not be quick to criticize. Patients may be reluctant to reveal their beliefs in folk medicine practices because they fear being ridiculed. And skepticism among physicians and dentists concerning the value of folk remedies will even cause individuals to avoid needed treatment. Therefore, harmless practices can be allowed to continue, but the patient should be taught alternative practices to potentially harmful customs. The patient should be taught to seek care for illness not amenable to folk remedy. Although most practices are harmless and may even provide a very beneficial placebo effect, the majority of cases in the literature that were wrongly suspected as child abuse involved vigorous overtreatment and abuses, not routine practices.

International Definition

To prevent false accusations of child abuse, practitioners will have to agree on a standard definition of child abuse that can be applied to all cultures. This is not an easy task from a cross-cultural perspective. Anthropological study has revealed wide variability in child-rearing practices (Korbin, 1977). This variability ranges from harsh physical sanction to total indulgence. The Paua tribe of New Guinea allows severence of the child's digit or earlobe for infraction of the rules. Also, insertion of sharp reeds into the nostrils and tongue to induce bleeding is part of their initiation rites. On the other hand, the Polynesian culture is widely known for its permissive attitudes concerning child rearing. Comparing practices among different cultures is difficult. It would seem unreasonable to accuse a Yoruba mother who practices scarification on her children of abuse when our culture sanctions orthodontic care and condones parental pressure on children to participate in athletics, which can terminate in injury. All three cultural practices can be painful to the child but are practiced in order to make the child more acceptable to other members of the culture.

Child-rearing practices must be viewed within their cultural contexts while still meeting some standard of international acceptability. Appropriate guidelines for the development of an international definition of child abuse should include: *(a)* a culturally relative outlook, *(b)* a universally humane standard, and *(c)* an opposition to imposing ethnocentric expectations (Korbin, 1977).

When developing an international definition of child abuse, the following contextual factors should be taken into account before a folk medicine practice is considered abusive (Korbin, 1977).

- Is the act accepted within the culture?
- Are there rules governing it, or is it an aberrant and idiosyncratic act in a culture that has no context for the behavior?
- How far does the act deviate from accepted standards of conduct within the culture?
- What is the intent of the act?
- What is the child's perception of the act?
- Is the act considered necessary for the successful maturation of the child by the culture?

Summary

Several folk medicine practices that closely mimic child abuse have been described. However, because these practices were performed according to well-accepted cultural beliefs, without malice, and in the context of true concern for the child's well-being, they should not be considered as child abuse nor should they be managed as such. The case reports in the literature represent overzealous treatment or misguided adherence to folk medicine beliefs.

When health professionals encounter folk medicine practices, they should not criticize or ridicule them, but rather extend suggestions for alternative measures. Since most folk beliefs are harmless, though deeply ingrained in tradition, they should be discussed in neutral terms in order to improve acceptance and compliance with modern health practices when truly needed. Hopefully, folk medicine beliefs will be better understood and managed through an internationally accepted definition of child abuse. Distress of parents falsely accused of child abuse could then be eliminated in the future.

References

Ahn, N.: ''Pseudo-battered Child'' Syndrome. J. Am. Med. Assoc. 236:2288, 1976.

Du, J.N.: Pseudobattered Child Syndrome in Vietnamese Immigrant Children. Can. Med. Assoc. J. 122:394, 1980.

Geffner, M.E. and Sandler, A.P.: Oral Metallic Mercury. A Folk Medicine Remedy for Gastroenteritis. Clin. Pediatr. 19:435, 1980.

Gellis, S.; Feingold, M.; Yeatman, M.; Shaw, C.; Barlow, M.; and Bartlett, G.: Picture of the Month—Cao Gio (Pseudobattering in Vietnamese Children). Am. J. Dis. Child 130:857–585, 1976.

Guarnaschelli, J.; Lee, J.; and Pitts, F.W.: ''Fallen Fontanelle'' (Caida de Mollera): A Variant of the Battered Child Syndrome. J. Am. Med. Assoc. 222:1545, 1972.

Ho-Quang-Phuoc, E.: Cao Gio—An Explanation. Personal Communication, 1981.

Hughes, W.T.: Superstitions and Home Remedies Encountered in Present Day Pediatric Practice in the South. J. Ky. State Med. Assoc. 61:25, 1963.

Keller, E.L. and Apthorp, J.: Folk Remedies vs. Child Battering. Am. J. Dis. Child 131:1173, 1977.

Keller, E.L. and Blair, J.: Folk Remedies. West. J. Med. 125:55, 1976.

Korbin, J.: Anthropological Contributions to the Study of Child Abuse. Child Abuse Neglect 1:7, 1977.

Primosch, R.E. and Young, S.K.: Pseudobattering of Vietnamese Children (Cao Gio). J. Am. Med. Assoc. 101:47, 1980.

Rubenstein, A.: Absence of Uvula in South Sinai Bedouins. J. Am. Med. Assoc. 242:323, 1979.

Sandler, A.P. and Chan, L.S.: Mexican-American Folk Belief in a Pediatric Emergency Room. Med. Care 16:778, 1978.

Sandler, A.P. and Haynes, V.: Nonaccidental Trauma and Medical Folk Belief: A Case of Cupping. Pediatrics 61:921, 1978.

Snow, L.F.: Folk Medical Beliefs and Their Implications for Care of Patients. A Review Based on Studies Among Black Americans. Ann. Intern. Med. 81:82, 1974.

Stoeckle, D.B. and Carter, R.D.: Cupping in New York State—1978. N.Y. State J. Med. 80:117–20, 1980.

Taylor, L. and Newberger, E.: Child Abuse in the International Year of the Child. New Eng. J. Med. 301:1205, 1979.

Time Inc.: Folk Remedy—Coin Rubbing Puzzles M.D.'s. Time, Dec. 29, 1980, p. 54.

Yeatman, G.W.: Cao Gio (Coin Rubbing)—Vietnamese Attitudes Toward Health Care. J. Am. Med. Assoc. 244:2748, 1980.

Yeatman, G.W.; Shaw, C.; Barlow, M.; and Bartlett, G.: Pseudobattering in Vietnamese Children. Pediatrics 58:616–618, 1976.

Chapter 16

Other Cultural Practices Suspected as Child Abuse

Ray E. Stewart

Introduction

Man is unique among earth creatures for his desires and attempts to alter natural body form and appearance. Evidence of alterations of physiogomy is found in several archeological and anthropological studies. Many of these practices have persisted with variation in modern society and provide the foundation for the billion-dollar worldwide cosmetic industry. Practices resulting in permanent alteration or deformation of body structures are relevant to health care professionals, and are of specific interest to the dentist when the altered structures are located in the head and neck regions.

When judging practices of body form alteration, it is essential to consider the socio-cultural environments in which they occur. What is customary and acceptable in one social or ethnic climate may be considered abusive and entirely unacceptable in another. Common folklore practices resulting in irreversible alteration of body form will be reviewed, with the socio-cultural origins of these practices emphasized.

In general, folklore practices are observed in preliterate, aboriginal societies but can persist as traditional or customary practices in semi-literate or lower socioeconomic segments of modern society. The spread of western civilization has led to the gradual disappearance and reduced prevalence of many such customs.

Foot Binding

One of the oldest known examples of body form alteration is foot binding, which results in gross deformation of the tarsal and metatarsal structures. Foot binding was practiced widely in China until as recently as the 1930s. As with many folklore practices, the active deformation is performed on only one sex—in this case, women. The custom is thought to have originated in ancient Chinese culture as a means of discouraging women from fleeing bondage, but over the centuries it has evolved into an effort to achieve a desirable cosmetic feature. In this context it is interesting to note the desire among modern women to have small feet.

Cranial Alteration

Artificial deformation of the cranium has been practiced by several societies and ethnic groups throughout history. Binding the heads of young children effectively redirects the dimensional changes normally occurring in the cranium to accommodate the growing brain. Two types of head deformation have been described (McGibbon, 1912): restrictive bindings can be placed to alter either anterior-posterior or circumferential dimensions.

Cranium binding has been observed in ancient Egyptians, Pacific Northwest Indians, and pre-Colombian Mezo-Americans (Oetterking, 1924; Haeberling and Gunther, 1930; Dingwall, 1931). Although these civilizations are widely separated by time, geography, and the levels of refinement and sophistication they have attained, this common practice raises speculation about possible past connections among them. Although performed now primarily for cosmetic reasons, the custom might have originated as a ritual to recreate the molding of the neonatal skull resulting from the birth process. Head binding could have assured an individual of being reborn into the afterlife more easily and less traumatically.

Skin Piercing

Numerous aboriginal groups in central and eastern Africa and in underdeveloped areas of South America continue to alter facial structures by piercing and stretching the earlobes, lips, and nostrils. The origin of these practices in certain societies remains speculative. Nose piercing and lip stretching were prevalent in warlike, belligerent societies, which could suggest they were adopted to impart an appearance of ferocity to intimidate adversaries. That the deformation was done primarily to adolescent males when they were expected to bear arms in times of aggression or defense further corroborates this theory. These practices now appear to be followed strictly for cosmetic purposes.

In its most minor form, piercing infant females' ears and placing various types of decorative earrings is widely practiced today in Central and North America. Although this practice rarely results in complications and morbidity, infections occasionally arise. This American version of piercing is also usually done without local anesthesia and for strictly cosmetic reasons.

Scarification and Tattooing

Widespread among many primitive and civilized societies, scarification and tattooing are means of beautification or adornment. Tattooing often expresses an individual's lifestyle or personality. Both scarification and tattooing have been employed by certain societies to establish the association or bondage of an individual to another person or group.

Tooth Extraction or Mutilation

Of particular interest to the dentist are folklore practices involving nontherapeutic extraction of teeth and alteration or mutilation of tooth form. The ritualistic extraction of one or more permanent teeth has been recorded in many primitive societies and has been practiced since prehistoric times. The origin and rationale of this custom remains speculative. It might have been adopted to insure the reincarnation of the individual by removing and preserving a durable portion of the body for use in the afterlife. The loss of a tooth, whether naturally or induced, was also equated to castration since the tooth was thought of as a sexual symbol. Nontherapeutic extraction of one or more teeth was also used by some societies as punishment for sexual perversities or indiscretions (Kanner, 1928). In one South Pacific society permanent incisors are extracted from adolescent females when they reach sexual maturity. Whether this custom was originally an initiation rite or a means of identifying a woman as fertile and capable of bearing children remains unknown. Most nontherapeutic extractions of teeth are parts of initiation ceremonies where a youth achieves full tribal membership, being reborn into a new environment and station within that society. The extraction of one or more permanent teeth is a ritualistic dramatization of the shedding of deciduous teeth and as such is an important part of the rebirth being celebrated by the initiation ceremony (Townend, 1963).

Extracting primary canines in children in certain African societies is an attempt to treat or alleviate febrile episodes. It is believed that by removing mandibular canines the source of fever has a means of exiting the body (Pindborg, 1969).

Many societies throughout history have altered normal tooth anatomy by filing and/or drilling with or without the placement of decorative inlaid materials. The custom was practiced in ancient Japanese society (Suzuki, 1940) and perhaps spread from Asia to the New World via the Bering Land Bridge. Tooth filing has been observed in skeletal remains recovered in Mexico and Central America dating to approximately 1400 to 1100 B.C. These same specimens often contained elaborate inlays and other decorative materials, especially in anterior teeth. The practice among some American blacks of placing gold inlays, gold crowns with windows, and even semi-precious stones on the facial surfaces of the anterior teeth could be a form of this custom. Tooth filing has been observed in certain black Caribbean cultures and is considered part of an attempt to resurrect old customs and traditions as a means of establishing tribal ties and influence.

Summary

Body form alterations deemed traditional, customary, and acceptable behavior in one society might be considered abusive in others. Conflicts and differences of opinion are to be expected wherever primitive and modern societies interface. Problems arise when the particular custom or practice is taken out of context and suspected to be abusive. An international definition of abuse and neglect as discussed in the preceding chapter is paramount to helping dentists avoid misdiagnosing a folklore practice as abuse.

References

Dingwall, E.J.: Artificial Cranial Deformation. London: John Bale Sons and Danielsson, 1931.

Haeberling, H. and Gunther, E.: Indians of Puget Sound, Publications of Anthropology. Seattle: University of Washington Press, 1930.

Kanner, L.: Folklore of the Teeth. New York: Macmillan, 1928.

McGibbon, H.: Artificially Deformed Skulls with Special Reference to the Temporal Bone and its Tympanic Portion. Laryngoscope 22:1165, 1912.

Oetteking, B.: Declination of the Basilaris in Normal and Artificially Deformed Skulls. Indian Notes and Monographs 27:3, 1924.

Pindborg, J.J.: Dental Mutilation and Associated Abnormalities in Uganda. Am. J. Phys. Anthropol. 31:383, 1969.

Suzuki, H.: Ueber 3 neue Funde der Zackenfeilung. J. Anthrop. Soc. Nippon 55:489, 1940.

Townend, B.R.: Non-therapeutic Extraction of Teeth and its Relation to the Ritual Disposal of Shed Deciduous Teeth. Br. Dent. J. 115:312, 354, 394, 1963.

Chapter 17

The Dentist as Child Abuser

Arthur J. Nowak

Introduction

Most children entering a dental office, whether for examination or preventive or restorative care, are cooperative. They can be separated from parents, adjust quickly to the dentist and dental auxiliaries, respond positively to requests made by the dentist during the appointment, tolerate injections, noises, and vibrations of the high-speed drill, and even depart with thanks and smile.

There are children, unfortunately, who are unwilling or unable to submit to dental procedures that are in their best interests. The reasons for the resistance or refusal to submit are varied and can include fear, stubbornness, lack of adequate information, a previous stressful experience, and/or a developmental disability. The dentist may also lack the experience of coping with such a child.

Management Techniques

A number of management techniques are available to reduce or eliminate the anxiety of these children, to lessen their physical resistance, and to improve their overall acceptance of dental treatment. These techniques are usually divided into nonpharmacotherapeutic and pharmacotherapeutic types (Wright, 1975).

Nonpharmacotherapeutic techniques include:

- Preappointment behavior modification, e.g., modeling
- Behavior shaping, e.g., tell-show-do
- Retraining methods, e.g., counseling and desensitization
- Restraining methods, e.g., oral props, body wraps, and aversive conditioning (hand-over-mouth)
- Adjunctive procedures, e.g., office design, apparel, scheduling, and auxiliaries
- Hypnosis
- Referral to a specialist

Pharmacotherapeutic techniques include:

- Oral, inhalation, intramuscular, intravenous, and rectal administration of drugs used in conscious sedation
- General anesthesia in the hospital
- Local anesthesia

When these techniques are used rationally by well-trained personnel with prior consultation and approval of the child's parents or guardians, the results are predictable and usually acceptable. The child's dental treatment is completed, future dental appointments are usually less anxiety-provoking, the child is not physically or emotionally harmed, and the parents are pleased with the results.

Unfortunately, occasions arise whereby the dentist and/or the auxiliary, because of frustrations, emotional distress, or temporary loss of professional demeanor, go beyond the recommended and acceptable limits of management techniques and place the child in a compromised, threatened, and defensive state. Physical, emotional, or sexual abuse can often result.

Concerns in Patient Management

Responsibility of the Health Professional

An abused child is one whose physical or mental welfare is harmed or threatened with harm by the acts or omissions of the parent or other person(s) responsible for the child's welfare. Harm in this definition refers to a number of situations including injuries that are inflicted or allowed to be inflicted as a result of excessive corporal punishment. Whether other persons responsible for the child's welfare include the health professional has not been determined. Nevertheless, when the parent is separated from the child and the child is being cared for by a health professional in a treatment area, the health professional is responsible for that child's welfare. Therefore, it seems appropriate that the laws that govern the parent or guardian with regard to abuse now protect the child from any harm or threatened harm by the health professional (Polier, 1975; USDHEW, 1975; Barowsky, 1976; Fisher et al., 1980).

Parental Consent

For the child who is unable or refuses to cooperate, the dentist must make a decision based on the circumstances of the situation and the resources available to him for patient management. As mentioned previously, many techniques commonly taught to dentists can assist in the management of an uncooperative child. The dentist must not only select the one most appropriate for the situation, but must also consult with the parent as to its use, its benefits, risks associated with it, results expected, and alternatives. The parent or guardian has the right to consent to the use of the technique or to refuse on behalf of the child.

Many dentists require standard consent forms be signed prior to treatment. Unfortunately, these consent forms usually are written in general terms and do not describe the management techniques that might be utilized. The courts have found these authorizations to be so ambiguous that they are completely worthless, and have held the practitioner liable for damages. The dentist should make every effort to explain to the parent the technique to be used and to obtain informed consent. Where problems have developed, lack of communication and understanding between the parent and dentist has been the factor most frequently mentioned (Sarner, 1963; Wood, 1967; Howard and Parks, 1973; Healy and Nowak, 1977; Morris, 1977).

Physical Contact

In the course of treatment the dentist and auxiliaries will make contact with the child. These contacts can be either incidental or intentional. The patient/parent gives consent to be touched by requesting an appointment and consenting to the examination either orally or in writing. This consent does not give the dentist or the auxiliary any special privileges beyond those that can reasonably be expected to be used during a routine examination. Nor does this consent give privilege to the dentist to apply corporal punishment—that is, spanking or slapping the minor patient. Any nonconsensual offensive touching is a battery, unless it is justified, for example, by self-defense. Thus, any sort of punitive slap or spanking can be a battery. The unconsented-to touching is a battery regardless of the amount of force used. The amount of force is, however, relevant to the determination of damages. The courts have indicated that the appropriateness of patient discipline will be measured by the necessity of force, the amount of the force, and the manner in which it is applied (Healy and Nowak, 1977).

Physical Discipline

To what extent parents may explicitly authorize others to discipline their children is controversial. When discipline is appropriate, the dentist should have the parent authorize him/her to exercise it. It is important that consent be received from the parent or guardian (Healy and Nowak, 1977).

Physical Restraint

Traditionally, physically restraining the uncooperative child can be done in conjunction with or after other management techniques. Physical restraint can vary from a gentle holding of the hands by the dental auxiliary to the use of body ties. Physical restraints have been used traditionally in medical practice to prevent minors from touching dressings or healing wounds, and/or to immobilize patients to prevent harm to the patient.

Disciplinary physical restraining in the dental office can be questionable. If the dental treatment is necessary and the dentist feels that it cannot be performed in any other manner, a physical restraint is clearly justifiable. However, if the procedure can safely be delayed until cooperation can be obtained, a restraint is less justifiable. Parents should be asked to authorize any physical restraints that are to be used to facilitate procedures that could be safely postponed (Healy and Nowak, 1977).

Aversive Conditioning

Another restraining technique can be used on an uncooperative child with whom communication cannot be established. It is commonly known in dentistry as the hand-over-mouth technique, but is more appropriately termed aversive conditioning. Normally used as a method of last resort, it is applied to obstreperous children 3 to 6 years old who have normal intelligence and communicative ability. It is not applied to children who are unable to cooperate because they are under sedation or have handicapping conditions.

Aversive conditioning is accepted by the profession but is not frequently employed. Without informed consent of the parent, the hand-over-mouth technique would be considered battery—the unprivileged touching of the body of another. Some practitioners have modified the original technique by not only placing the hand over the mouth but also closing off the airway by pinching the nose. Parents who have unexpectedly witnessed this technique or were informed of its use later by the child have expressed concern about its intensity and probable physical and/or psychological harm to the child who feels he/she might soon suffocate (Healy and Nowak, 1977).

Pharmacological Approaches

Pharmacological approaches to child management are usually chosen to reduce pain and immobilize the patient. Additional risks are introduced into the management routine when drugs are used. Parents should be advised thoroughly and given specific indications of any potential hazards and complications, the results expected, and any alternatives available (Wright, 1975).

Problems of Management Techniques

Problems with traditionally available management techniques center around their acceptability, their reasonableness, and a standard of care. Considerable confusion continues regarding the legality of management methods in relation to specific dental treatments. Dentists have an ethical responsibility to render care and to determine whether care should be rendered, yet they also have a legal responsibility to observe the full breadth of the patient's rights. This often must be done without a clear understanding of the legal implications of treatment or of the leanings of society and the courts. In this age of societal awareness in the area of abuse, the dentist is confronted with additional concerns in the management of patients who are uncontrollable or who resist treatment.

Complaints and/or Litigations

Complaints and/or litigation against dentists over the use of management techniques in uncooperative children are difficult to document. Computerized medi-

Table 17-1 States reporting and number of complaints

	Peer review	State boards of examiners
States	31 (62%)	29 (58%)
Reporting period (months)	12–30	12–114
Number of complaints	11	44

Table 17-2 Incidents that prompted complaint

	Peer review	State boards of examiners
Physical restraint	2	7
Hitting/slapping	1	11
Misuse/drug overuse	3	4
Offensive language	3	4
Inappropriate gestures	1	3

colegal literature searches and reports from the American Dental Association's By-Laws and Judicial Affairs Council revealed no formal complaints or litigations against dentists.

State Dental Peer Review Committees and State Boards of Dental Examiners did reveal significant findings when asked for information on complaints or incidents involving dentists and management of pediatric patients. The State Peer Review Committees, a mechanism within the dental profession since 1975, provides an expert and credible system for resolving disagreements that cannot be resolved at an earlier informal stage about the appropriateness and quality of care a dentist renders. The committee is appointed by the state society and is composed of well-respected practitioners in the state. Complaints registered against a practitioner can be presented to the committee, which through mediation attempts to resolve the differences between the patient/parent and the dentist. The committee has no disciplinary powers, but it can refer a case to an appropriate state agency. It is not within the committee's scope to consider cases in litigation. State Boards of Dental Examiners are charged to license dentists within their state and to monitor the affairs of those licensed dentists in protection of the consumer. The boards usually are informed of any complaints or litigation against dentists within the state.

Because it is impossible to determine whether the reports for the State Peer Review Committees and the State Board of Dental Examiners included the same complaints, these reports are discussed separately. The responses from the two groups were similar, with 31 or 62% of the committees responding and 20 or 58% of the boards responding (see Table 17-1). The reporting period varied from 12 to 30 months for the committees to 12 to 114 months for the boards (see Table 17-1). The number of complaints was low: 11 complaints have been reported and reviewed by the committees and 44 by the boards (see Table 17-1).

Table 17-3 Disposition of incidents

	Peer review	State boards of examiners
Physical injury	2	1
Death	0	1
Assault and battery		
DDS	0	6
Auxiliary	0	1
Litigation	3	4

No one type of incident seemed to be more likely to prompt complaints, although physical restraint (including hand-over-mouth) and hitting/slapping were reported more frequently than the misuse of drugs, offensive language, and inappropriate gestures. Unfortunately, 15 of the 44 complaints to the State Boards of Dental Examiners did not state the incident that prompted the complaint (see Table 17-2).

Information about the final dispositions of the incidents is limited. Nevertheless, the number of complaints that prompted litigation included three for the committees and four for the boards. Seven of the incidents reported to the boards resulted in assault and battery charges against the dentists or auxiliaries (see Table 17-3).

The State Boards of Dental Examiners data reported a higher number of female (14) than male (9) patients abused. The information from the State Peer Review Committees revealed little difference (see Table 17-4). The most cases reported by boards were in the 3- to 9-year age range (16), while in the committees no clear difference was reported (see Table 17-4). The State Boards of Dental Examiners information revealed the highest number of most adult abusers were in the 30- to 40-year group according to the boards, while the committees noted no clear difference (see Table 17-5). The sex of the abuser was overwhelmingly male in both groups (see Table 17-5). The general practitioner was involved more frequently in incidents reported to both the committees and the Boards (see Table 17-4). No data were received on any complaints suggesting sexual abuse between the dentist and the pediatric patient.

From the data reported, it is obvious that few complaints are reported to the committees and boards. The incidence of child abuse by the dental professional may be much higher than this indicates, but because of reporting mechanisms, complaints management, and confidentiality, it is impossible to determine the actual number. Most parents do not know the mechanisms available to them to register a complaint, and so rarely proceed any further than voicing their concern to the receptionist or the dentist. Often the child is taken to a different dentist for additional care.

When concern proceeds beyond discussion with the dentist and parent, legal counsel becomes involved and the negotiations continue with the insurance carrier. Results are confidential, making it impossible to document the magnitude of alleged child abuse by dental practitioners.

Table 17-4 Ages and sexes of abused patients

	Peer review	State boards of examiners
Age (years)		
0–3	0	2
3–6	3	9
6–9	1	7
9–12	2	2
>12	2	2
Sex		
Male	4	9
Female	3	14

Table 17-5 Ages, sexes, and practice designations of abusers

	Peer review	State boards of examiners
Age (years)		
<30	0	1
30–40	5	10
40–50	3	4
50–60	0	2
>60	0	2
Sex		
Male	8	18
Female	0	0
Designation		
GP	5	12
Specialist	3	5

From the little data reported, it appears that physical restraint and corporal punishment cause most complaints. What happens between the defiant and uncooperative patient and the dentist and/or auxiliary to lead to excessive force and physical punishment can only be speculated. Anger, fear, professional pride, ego, frustration, and/or the inability to cope with the child are all implicated.

Because battery, the unprivileged touching of another's body, was the most frequent formal accusation reported, it is important for the dentist to review with parents the management techniques he/she proposes to use and to either receive informed consent, delay treatment, or refer completion of treatment to a specialist. The parents most often had not been informed of the technique used, and if they had been, they reportedly would probably not have registered complaints.

Summary

Although there are evidence of and concern over physical child abuse by dental professionals, the techniques utilized in the dentist's office to manage a defiant and uncooperative child have been little-discussed. There have been occasional reports of complaints registered by parents on techniques used by dentists, but documentation fails to provide accurate incidence data. Although the incidence of reported physical child abuse in the dental office appears low, the actual incidence may be greater.

The following recommendations for the dental profession seem appropriate:

- Before treating a child a dentist should inform the parents or guardians of the procedures and techniques that will be used and should obtain informed consent for these.
- If it is anticipated that the child will be defiant and uncooperative, the dentist might suggest to the parents or guardians that treatment be delayed or referred, especially if delay will not jeopardize the health or the final outcome of treatment.
- If treatment cannot be delayed or referred, the dentist should explain to the parents the management technique to be used, emphasizing the risks and benefits as well as the alternatives. Consent should be expressed and informed. Blanket consents in broad and general terms may be more dangerous than no consent at all.
- If during a management session it becomes apparent that the child cannot be managed, and the dentist and/or auxiliary are becoming frustrated or angry, it is best that the treatment be discontinued and alternative choices considered. If none is available, he or she should consult with the parents or guardians and recommend alternatives.
- More thorough documentation of complaints is needed to study the variety of management techniques. State Boards of Dental Examiners, State Peer Review Committees, and Professional Liability Insurance carriers should be encouraged to register complaints and litigations and to provide them to behavior scientists so that management techniques and their applications in dental practice can be comprehensively reviewed by the dental and legal professions.

References

Barowsky, E.I.: The Abuse and Neglect of Handicapped Children by Professionals and Parents. J. Pediatr. Psych. 1:44, 1976.

Fisher, B.; Berdie, J.; Cook, J.; and Day, N.: Adolescent Abuse and Neglect, Intervention Strategies. U.S. Dep. of Health and Human Services Pub. No. (OHDS) 80-30266, Washington, D.C., 1980.

Healy, A. and Nowak, A.: Management of Children by Health Professionals. Iowa City: University of Iowa Press, 1977.

Howard, W. and Parks, A.: The Dentist and the Law. (3rd Ed.). St. Louis: C.V. Mosby, 1973.

Morris, W.O.: Dental Litigation. (2nd Ed.). Charlottesville: The Miche Co., 1977.

Polier, H.J.: Professional Abuse of Children: Responsibility for the Delivery of Services. Am. J. Orthopsych. 45:357, 1975.

Sarner, H.: Dental Jurisprudence. Philadelphia: W.B. Saunders, 1963.

Wood, L.B.: A Handbook of Dental Malpractice. Springfield: C.C. Thomas, 1967.

Wright, G.Z.: Behavior Management in Dentistry for Children. Philadelphia: W.B. Saunders, 1975.

U.S. Department of Health, Education and Welfare: Child Abuse and Neglect: The Problem and Its Management. Vol. 1, An Overview of the Problem. HEW Pub. No. (OHD) 75-30073, Washington, D.C., 1975.

Chapter 18

A Case of Child Abuse

Richard S. Sobel
David L. Kerns

A four-year-old black male was presented by his mother to Children's Hospital Medical Center of Northern California Dental Service with a chief complaint of injuries secondary to a fall at home. Injuries included oral facial lacerations, bruises, and displaced primary teeth.

Health History

The child was apparently healthy, and had a medical history characterized by irregular and inconsistent pediatric care. An interview with the mother revealed that two hours before he had fallen at home and had hit his face against a table. He reportedly had been playing with a toy, and no adult was present when the injury occurred. He suffered intraoral bleeding and displaced teeth.

Oral Facial Examination

Oral facial examination revealed several older facial abrasions and bruises that were healing normally. Recent injuries included bruised upper and lower lips and a 3.4-centimeter bruise on the chin. Intraoral examination revealed lacerations of the maxillary anterior gingiva and alveolar mucosa. Intrusion of the primary left maxillary lateral incisor had occurred and the primary left maxillary central incisor was absent (Fig. 18-1). Multiple carious lesions were presented with no evidence of dental care. Oral hygiene was poor. All bruised areas were tender when palpated, especially those adjacent to the intruded tooth and the mandible. The anterior portion of the mandible was slightly mobile when palpated.

Intraoral Radiographic Survey

Intraoral radiographic survey verified the intrusion of the primary left maxillary lateral incisor and avulsion of the primary left maxillary central incisor. Occlusal radiographic survey revealed a fracture of the mandible between the central and lateral incisors (Fig. 18-2).

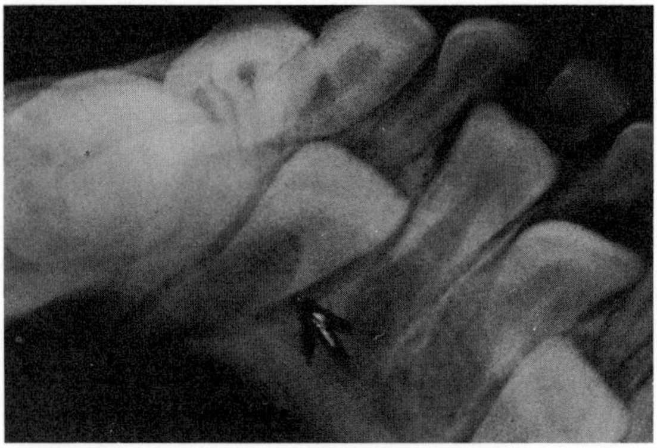

Fig. 18-1 Intraoral appearance revealing lacerations of the gingiva and intrusion of the primary maxillary lateral incisor and avulsion of the maxillary left central incisor.

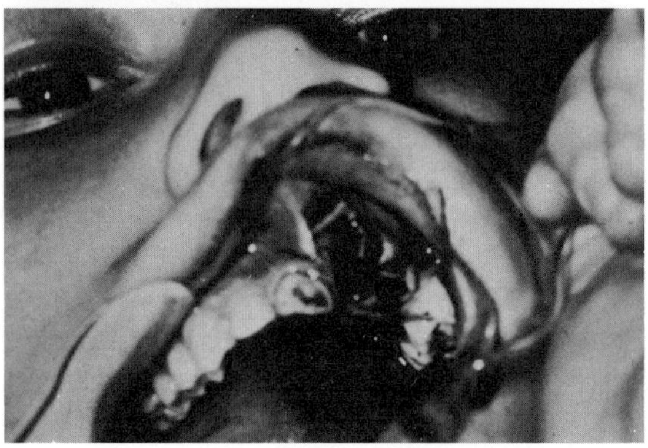

Fig. 18-2 Intraoral radiograph depicting fracture of the mandible between the central and lateral incisors.

The serious, multiple injuries were disproportionate to those that could result from a moderately traumatic event. The bruises were in different stages of healing and lesions had apparently occurred over a period of time. Consent, although not legally necessary, was obtained for facial and intraoral photography. The mother was questioned further about previous and current injuries.

Treatment

The intraoral lesions were debrided and stabilized and the patient was referred to the Emergency Medical Service for a thorough physical evaluation. The suspicious nonaccidental injuries in the oral facial region and on the upper extremities, and the seriousness of these injuries, dictated such a referral immediately.

Physical Examination and Laboratory Data

Physical examination revealed multiple bruises predominantly on the back and the right arm that varied from reddish-purple to brown, with many having "loop-mark" patterns (Figs. 18-3 and 18-4). In addition, there were circular, healing

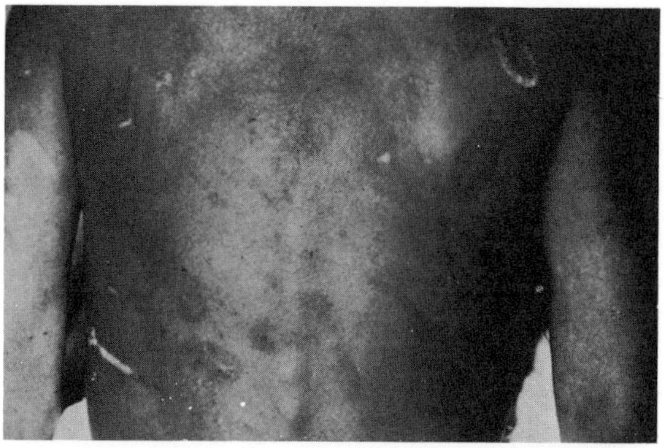

Fig. 18-3 Patient's back revealing bruises from belt loops.

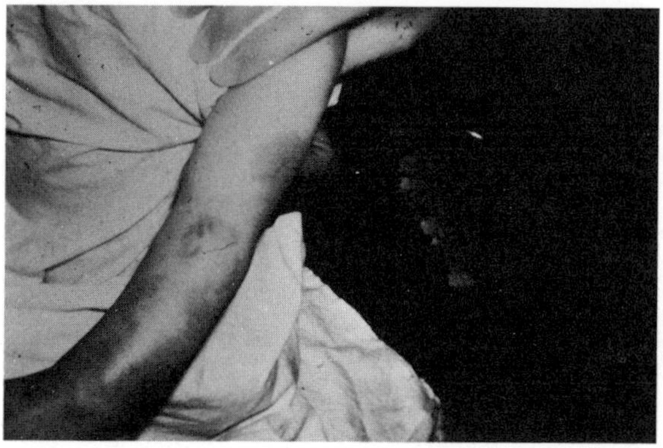

Fig. 18-4 Patient's right arm with multiple bruise marks.

lesions resembling healing cigarette burns on the palms of both hands (Fig. 18-5). The remainder of the physical examination was unremarkable.

Radiographs of the skull, long bones, ribs, and pelvis were within normal limits. A coagulation screen including platelet count, prothrombin time, and partial thromboplastin time was normal.

Parent Counseling

The parent was informed of the suspicion regarding the multiple injuries and was requested to meet with a social worker. During this interview the following psychosocial history was obtained. The father and mother had been living together for approximately eight years and had two other children, ages seven years and 10 months. The father had been regularly employed until recently, but was currently unemployed. He was a chronic alcoholic and on a number of occasions had physically abused both the children and his spouse. The mother appeared passive and ineffectual during the interview. She acted in an immature manner in response to family issues. Apparently the father often acted in a similar manner.

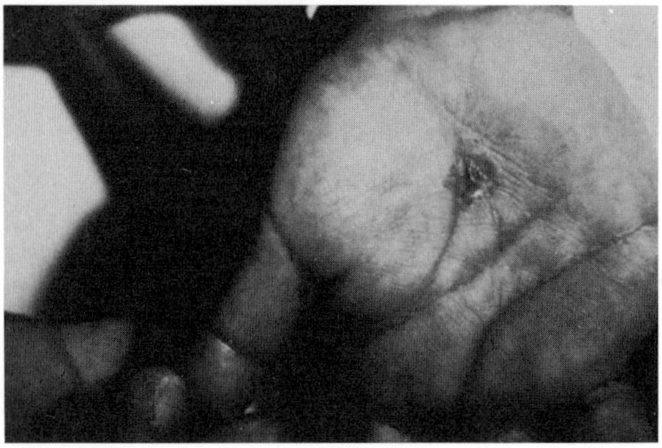

Fig. 18-5 Palmar aspect of hand—healing cigarette burn.

Protective Services

The social worker, physician, and dentist discussed the reportability of this suspicious incident in light of their mutual findings and the risk of the child being injured again. Taken into account were the child's age, the psychosocial history of the family, and the severity, number, and types of injuries, especially those most recently occurring to the head.

The group decided to hospitalize the child with the admitting diagnosis of "unexplained injuries." The parents were notified by the physician of the decision to admit the child and of the necessity of reporting the occurrence to child protective services. They were reassured that the professionals involved would work with the family to find better methods for the parents to deal with their child.

Reporting

Telephone and written reports to child protective services were made. These included:

- Demographic information, including patient and parent name and address
- Time, day, and date of presentation
- History, including detailed sequence of events, discovery of the injury, and the persons present at the time of injury
- Detailed physical findings, including characteristics, color, and location of each individual lesion
- Results of radiographic and laboratory tests
- Conclusion stating that the incident appeared to represent nonaccidental trauma and evaluating the risk of reinjury to the child

Hospital Course

During the child's 72-hour hospital stay dental care was continued and supportive medical care was delivered. Developmental screening revealed deficiencies in language development. Both siblings were given physical examinations, which revealed no evidence of trauma or injury. Developmental screening revealed a mild language delay in the seven-year-old. She was also immature in her interactions with adults.

The child protective services worker interviewed both parents extensively. The parents refused voluntary foster placement of the four-year-old child. Child protective services, therefore, obtained temporary custody pending a hearing before the Juvenile Court and placed him in a foster home. Since no evidence of physical abuse was found for the other siblings, they were allowed to remain in the natural home.

Legal Proceedings

Before appearing in court the physician, dentist, and child protective services worker needed to prepare evidence and testimony. A pretrial conference was arranged since this was the first appearance for the dentist before the Juvenile Court. All dental, medical, and protective service records were reviewed in an informal discussion with the county attorney, which helped each of the professionals to become more familiar with issues relevant to the court hearing.

As expert witnesses, the physician and dentist were asked to testify on specific matters in the case and to answer questions related to hypothetical situations regarding the child and his suspected abuse. They were asked questions that explored the patient's examination, circumstances of the examination, presence of other people at the examination, the history taken from parents, and specifically the nature and extent of the injuries, their causes, and prognosis. Interpretations of radiographic and laboratory findings were reviewed.

The court ruled that there was sufficient evidence to support the allegation of child physical abuse. It elected to place the child in foster care for a minimum of six months. During this placement, medical and dental treatment were to be continued for resolution of all physically traumatized areas. Frequent visits by the child protective services worker would monitor the progress of the child in physical and emotional recovery.

Parental Therapy

In addition to the foster placement, the following therapy plan was developed for the family:

- The mother and father were referred for weekly marital/family counseling.
- Both parents would join the local Parents Anonymous chapter.
- The 10-month-old sibling would enter a day care center three afternoons per week.
- The father was referred to Alcoholics Anonymous.
- The family was referred to a public assistance social worker in the Department of Social Services for support during periods of financial need.
- Both the patient and his seven-year-old sibling were referred for speech and language therapy.

The court encouraged parental visitation twice weekly while their son was in foster care. There was also agreement that after a six-month period of therapy, the family's progress would be reviewed and the return of the child would be considered by the court.

Case Resolution

During the next six months the parents both complied with their marital/family therapy appointments as well as their Parents Anonymous activities. The father regularly attended Alcoholics Anonymous meetings for three months and became employed in the community. The mother stated that she and her husband were benefiting from both their psychotherapy and their Parents Anonymous experience. After case review, the child protective services agency felt that it was appropriate to return the child to the natural home under continuing child protective supervision by their agency.

Summary

An exemplary case of child physical abuse presenting to a dental office has been presented. Since child physical abuse encompasses health, social, and legal issues, the case was reviewed with these aspects emphasized by diagnosis and treatment. All issues must, however, be attended to with equal thrust and direction for successful case resolution.

Reference

U.S. Department of Health, Education and Welfare: Child Abuse and Neglect: The Problem and Its Management. Vol. 1, An Overview of the Problem. HEW Pub. No. (OHD) 75-30073, Washington, D.C., 1975.

Index